Praise for *Swaddled*

"*Swaddled* is a much-needed salve for the new mother. Through honest sharing and raw storytelling, Cassidy tenderly holds our hand and walks us through what it truly *feels* like to be a new mother. A transition that forever changes us, and only for the better, when we learn how to care for ourselves and each other in the process."

—Amy Owen, yoga instructor and birth coach

"How do you learn to mother? Whether you are already a mother or about to become one, the mothers who speak to you through *Swaddled* reach out with guidance and kind encouragement. Read their stories, absorb their support, and pass it on. Mothering is an ancient human task, and as stated by one mother in the book, 'I actually don't think anyone is meant to mother alone.'"

—Ann Jordahl, counselor and parent-infant instructor

"Finally, a book offering moms and their loved ones a genuine understanding of the bliss *and* the unexpected turmoil of pregnancy, birth, and early motherhood. Cassidy shines a light on the emotional rollercoaster of matrescence—the insecurity, loneliness, grief, and ambivalence—that many mothers experience. This empowering story collection helps prepare women for both the joys and the tribulations of early motherhood, while modeling a pathway for resilience, connection, and personal growth."

—Angele Close, PhD, clinical psychologist

"What a beautiful gift to know I'm not alone in my struggles as a new mama."

—Malia, stay-at-home mother of two

"*Swaddled* brings an important, moving and relatable message to the world of new motherhood. I saw in the stories that are so lovingly shared the experiences of many of my therapy clients, who feel guilt, shame and loneliness when their lived experience as a new mother does not match the image projected by society. It also reminded me of my own experiences as a mother; that it can be and is hard, that we all need community and connection, and that the challenges are temporary and ever-changing. A must read for all new mothers, and for those supporting and loving them."

—Noelle McWard Aquino, LCSW,
psychotherapist and author of
Anxiety Unpacked: Discover Your Type and Recover Your Peace

"This is the book I needed when I had my first child. I wish I'd had the embrace of knowing I wasn't alone in my self-doubt and fear of being a new mother. *Swaddled* is a game changer, opening the conversation about what it really looks like to become the lifeline for the most important—and entirely dependent—person in the world, your baby . . . when there's no room for error and you've never done the job before."

—Denise, working mother of two

"Life-altering honesty in ditching the comparison game and respecting yourself as the perfect mother to your child, regardless of how anyone else does motherhood."

—Ella, stay-at-home mother of four

"A healing read for every mother: new mothers in the trenches and those who've survived to thrive and look back with sweet nostalgia or maybe even a little doubt or confusion."

—Camile, working mother of one

Swaddled

Swaddled

Sage Stories to Wrap Mothers in Love

ELIZABETH SARAH CASSIDY

STARLING
PRESS

Swaddled: Sage Stories to Wrap Mothers in Love
Published in the United States by Starling Press, Illinois.

Copyright ©2025 by Elizabeth Sarah Cassidy

All rights reserved. No part of this book may be reproduced in any form or by any mechanical means, including information storage and retrieval systems without permission in writing from the publisher/author, except by a reviewer who may quote passages in a review. All images, logos, quotes, and trademarks included in this book are subject to use according to trademark and copyright laws of the United States of America.

Cassidy, Elizabeth Sarah, Author
Swaddled
Elizabeth Sarah Cassidy

Library of Congress Control Number 2025902920

ISBN 979-8-9926413-0-1, 979-8-9926413-2-5 (paperback)
ISBN 979-8-9926413-3-2 (hardcover)
ISBN 979-8-9926413-1-8 (digital)

FAMILY & RELATIONSHIPS / Parenting / Motherhood
HEALTH & FITNESS / Pregnancy & Childbirth
BODY, MIND & SPIRIT / Inspiration & Personal Growth
MEDICAL / Nursing / Maternity, Perinatal, Women's Health

Book interior design by Claudine Mansour Design
Publishing Management: Susie Schaefer, Finish the Book Publishing

Quantity Purchases: Schools, companies, professional groups, clubs, and other organizations may qualify for special terms when ordering quantities of this title. For information, email info@starling-press.com.

All rights reserved by Elizabeth Sarah Cassidy and Starling Press
Printed in the United States of America

*Dedicated to my father, Philip Justin Smith,
for naming me Elizabeth Sarah instead of
Sarah Elizabeth because it would look better on a
book cover one day.*

*And to my mother, Carol Ann Smith, for agreeing to the
name and for being one of the strongest people I know.*

*This is for both of you.
Thank you for inspiring this work and the support
I hope it will provide to many women.*

Motherhood's Contradiction

by Jessica Urlichs, featured in *All I See is You*

I've been the happiest since I've had children.
I've also been at my lowest.

I'm a much better version of myself.
I also haven't always liked what I've seen when mirrors have been held up to me.

I've never been in more company.
And at times never felt so lonely.

Some days I don't want to end.
Some days I wish away, oh and the guilt from feeling that when they grow so fast.

I've never been so sure of who I'm meant to be.
I've never wondered so much who I am.

I've never felt closer with my husband.
But at times, I've never felt more distant.

I believe in myself, I trust myself.
I've questioned myself and doubted myself.

I always want to be better for them.
But I've yelled and cried and wished I'd handled certain situations better.

I've never loved so hard and so fiercely.
And I've never felt so vulnerable.

I've never been more broken.
And I've never been more complete.

I've never smiled so much.
I've never cried so much.

I've never craved alone time more.
But when I am I always feel like something's missing, like an arm.

I've never been so excited to watch them grow.
And simultaneously wished they'd stay little forever.

Some days I feel like I've achieved nothing.
But as I think of them at night, I know I've achieved everything.
I've never looked forward to so much.
And I've also, never looked back.

It's one beautiful contradiction.
A journey of wrong turns that are probably still right.
And dreams of the future even if you don't get enough sleep to dream.
Exhaustion but effortless love.
The hardest and most rewarding thing ever.
Motherhood.

Contents

Preface No One Told Me — xiii

1. Lifelines — 1
   MY STORY

2. Fab Four — 25
   DANIELLE

3. Clueless with a Capital "C" — 41
   MONICA

4. Bikinis, Barbies, and Christmas Pizza — 59
   AIMEE

5. To Thine Own Self be True — 79
   SARA

6. Amazing Grace — 91
   SHERYL

7. The Married Single Mom — 107
   BRIE

8. Doctor's Orders — 127
   MEREDITH

9. The Gift of Signs — 145
   NICOLE

10.	**Close Call** CORA	165
11.	**Flow** AMANDA	175
12.	**Red Rope** ASHLEE	191

Epilogue **Matrescence and Me**	207
Closing **Your Story**	211
Acknowledgments	213
Playlist	217
About the Author	219

Preface

No One Told Me

"'Child,' said the Lion, 'I am telling you your story, not hers. No one is told any story but her own.'"

—C.S. Lewis, *The Horse and His Boy*

I wrote this book because no one told me. No one told me how it would be to be a new mother, particularly a first-time mother. How it would be . . . *really*. And once I was in the enormity of new motherhood, no one told me that my life would eventually come back to me. Not my friends, not my grandmother, not my aunts, not my mother-in-law, not even my own mother. I'm not mad at these ladies; I learned long ago that grudges aren't the way to go. However, perhaps if someone had issued some gentle foresight and hopeful assurance before and after the big pop, I could have avoided some pretty dark days.

Even if I didn't fully embrace the assurances as truth at the time, I could have held that hope in the back of my mind . . . or in any part of my body. Instead, I had no hope. My early days as a mama were bleak, as I mourned my prior existence and saw no path to success with my new job as a mother. How sad, how unnecessary, and how avoidable. The thought that I could help other women, save them from similar struggle, didn't hit me until well after I welcomed my third son, about six years after the surprise news that I was expecting my first.

You see, there was a significant gap between the vision that society sold me about motherhood and what those early days and months were actually like. They weren't the magic I had been promised by greeting cards, baby showers, advertisements, and television. A delusion. If those outlays reflected real life accurately, no one would watch them, no one would buy them. Further, if they were honest renditions, women around the world might not ever "pull the goalie," so to speak. After all, how does anyone ever indubitably know that she's ready to entirely upend her life? Perhaps motherhood's eradication of everything a woman knows as normal is a secret kept unconsciously to protect the species' propagation. I'm kidding, kind of.

I believe both realities can be true: that new motherhood is wonderful and that it's hard. Let's not skirt the hard. Let's be honest. Let's be real. I expect there are women out there whose experiences are, in fact, consistent with their social media accounts: those with radiant, cosmetically enhanced faces, tightly embraced by partners espousing deep, honeymoon-esque love, angelic babies (without a hint of baby acne), and zero crying (by anyone involved). And that's great! I'm not bitter. I've made it a policy to renounce bitterness, just as I do grudges. We should be happy for these successful, enamored, and fulfilled women. We *are* happy for them, but there is great variability across new mothers' experiences. At one end of the spectrum are the mothers lucky enough to have delivered perfect, healthy babies who sleep through the night from the get-go and who rarely shriek like banshees. These mothers' nerves are mostly intact, and they continue on their life's trajectory without too much turbulence. At the other end of the spectrum are the mothers who have serious pregnancy complications, suffer postpartum depression, or whose babies require life-sustaining medical interventions. Their babies are perfect, too, by the way. These mothers can experience a deep sense of turmoil and often feel disoriented in their suddenly new circumstances. And there's a whole lot of gray space in between those extremes as illustrated in the stories of this book.

I wrote *Swaddled* to open the conversation about what it's *really* like to be a new mama ... with no job experience. Indeed, it's tremendously joyful, promising, and awe-inspiring. But it's also scary, it's f'ing hard, it's lonely at times, and it can rock you to your core. New motherhood is many different things to each woman who embarks on this remarkable, life-altering journey. Let's celebrate that. Let's say it the way it is, and let's support each other.

Facades come easily to me. In the past, my perception of how others believed I should live drove my behavior. It was innocent enough, a people-pleasing move. Yet, I can see where some might call me an A+ liar, an impostor. I didn't intend to deceive, but rather, it was a protection mechanism. People thought I was competent, satisfied, secure, and what *they* thought was more important to me than how *I* felt. I stuffed my feelings, and this tendency flared at my entrance to motherhood. Specifically, I feigned an effortless adjustment. All was well, I was fine, everything was fine.

What is abundantly clear to me is that we need to get more comfortable asking for help. And asking for help is easier under perfect conditions, like when we're explicitly asked if we need help. Because some of us put on a really good act, it's important to check on our friends. We don't truly know how someone is doing unless we dare to ask. Even when we do ask, sometimes we need to ask the next question and then the next. Go deeper because it's easier to tell the truth when prompted to do so. Glennon Doyle, someone I strongly admire for her brave capacity to live her truth, says, "People who need help sometimes look a lot like people who don't need help." There are many variations on this concept, but the idea is to proactively check in with your strong friend, your busy friend, your "happy" friend . . . you know, the ones who seem to handle everything (including motherhood) so very well. Let's give mothers the opportunity to ditch the disguise and be real.

Let's be the people who want to hear the truth because the truth is liberating and empowering . . . for both the speaker and the listener. Someone has to be willing to listen, but first, someone needs to risk telling the truth in order to ask for help. Only in community can we experience the tribe of motherhood in its full glory, and only through exposure to how things really are can we find genuine connection. Truth vibrates for everyone's benefit.

What follows is meant to be an ultimately honest, and at times lightly humorous, glimpse at the vulnerability and drama of new motherhood. It's based on reality, not what society purports as the exultations of new motherhood. There is, in fact, joy involved, but it comes along with (and sometimes after) a bunch of other stuff. The dynamics of judgment, comparison, and perfectionism rear their ugly faces everywhere for new mothers. Even so, we're expected to sentimentalize the experience, which is often impossible in light of sleep deprivation, physical recovery, emotional stress, and so much more.

In the same way babies receive comfort and security when swaddled, so too do new mothers require such embrace during this tumultuous time. *Swaddled* is a heartwarming compilation of women finding survival, solace, and confidence, often in the arms and stories of other women. The accounts herein are all based on real women, although some names, identifying characteristics, locations and timeframes have been changed to protect the privacy of the people involved.

These women represent only a small slice of the population of mothers. Not everyone will experience what these ladies have, of course, and it would be impossible to incorporate every potential experience. Even if your specific circumstance isn't illustrated herein, my hope is that you'll feel the connection, depth, and oneness of the uniquely profound experience of new motherhood. It was an immense privilege to speak to these ladies, some still in the throes of their stories, some decades out of theirs. My respect and admiration for their core wisdom, strength, and life-giving energy is beyond words. Literally.

There are books that serve as instruction manuals for pregnancy and Baby's first year. But these aren't survival guides for the heart. For example, how are you supposed to feel if things don't go according to the literature? We might feel different, guilty, or ashamed. We might construe ourselves to, in fact, be a failure if our stories don't match what is said to be customary. But what or whose metrics of success are we using to determine our own sense of worth as mothers? What would happen if we dropped the comparison game and honored what is uniquely right for each of us as mothers and for our babies?

This book is in your hands for a reason. You're meant to ingest what these pages hold and represent, and I hope you'll share them with others. You know your baby, and you inherently and intuitively know how to care for your baby. You are a good mother. You know what to do and how to do it in a way that's exactly right for your baby . . . and YOU.

As women, and as mothers in particular, we never stop analyzing and assessing. We critique ourselves, and we critique others. Oftentimes, our own performance as mothers is the subject of our self-judgment and criticism. Other times, we evaluate how other women mother their children. This happens both consciously and unconsciously. Regardless of when you were a new mother, I hope this book brings compassion, catharsis, and community . . . to you and the mothers you know and love. I hope it heals.

We mothers are all in this together. Our circumstances vary widely, but in our unconditional love for our children and our personal evolutions, we are one. From these pages, I'm sending you tremendous love and so much respect and admiration. Congratulations on your motherhood. Your story is your story because it was meant to go down as it did. You are the perfect mother to your child or children. You represent the epitome of love. You are worthy. You *are* love, and I love you for it.

No one told me. So, I'm telling you. You are not alone. You're not the only one who has these feelings. Your life will come back to you, albeit in a different way: a bigger and better way. Yes, there will be bumps along the way, but there are ways over and around the bumps . . . especially when we mothers link arms, listen to one another, try to understand, and share our real stories.

Swaddled

Chapter 1

Lifelines

MY STORY

> *"I dare you to take off the mask of perfection and show up as you are. Feel the freedom, the relief, the lightness. Because when we are real, that's when we actually heal. And those around us just might heal, too."*
> —Ashley Hetherington

Chicago, October 7th

Dear Dad,

Thank you for the dream, the monarch, the deer . . . all the signs. I sure do miss you, our daily chats, and pondering life together. It's not fair that my baby won't know his Grandpa Phil. Sometimes, I get angry, and when I do, I hold tight to the magic of the Universe delivering me a new best friend . . . exactly a year after my first one was taken away. I feel your hand in this, Dad.

You'd laugh if you saw me right now. People tell me I don't look pregnant from behind, a big compliment. But from any other angle, I'm about to burst. I think you'd be proud of how I've prepared for this little guy, just like you taught me. There's always more to learn, but I've read three shelves worth of parenting books. I'm out of space. The nursery is stocked, and his clothes are organized by function then color. The 529 account is ready to be funded. Every to-do is crossed off, and I can't even think of another list to write. I've transitioned my clients and recently won another award for exceeding my sales quota. You've always supported my work and my success, and I hope I can make you proud as a mother.

It's all done, and I'm ready! I've got this; stay tuned.

Love,
Lizzy Sarah

Ryan Philip entered this world two days later and one week before my 28th birthday. At 9 pounds, 2 ounces, 21.5 inches (significantly larger than predicted), he didn't come flying out of my petite frame. The forceps and vacuum couldn't prevent his shoulder from getting stuck. The delivery quickly escalated to an emergency requiring the troops to be called in. Deaf to my screams to push him back up and cut him out, one of the doctors climbed on top of me and pushed. Another had her hands, forearms, and elbows inside me to manipulate Ryan from my war-torn birth canal. It wasn't the experience I had trained for with my doula. So much for the essential oils, breathwork, and yoga squats. There was no spa music after all.

I didn't get to hold him right away because the doctors whisked him off. He passed all the critical tests, but his right arm was immobile. The doctors assured me that the nerve damage was temporary. I cradled him like a China doll when I was finally permitted to hold my baby. His rough ride left him looking like he'd been in a back-alley brawl. One eye was swollen shut, his face was lopsided, and his head was shaped like an egg. I focused on his very long fingers, innocent eyes, and hair that fell just over his ears. There we were, two banged-up Libras smitten to finally meet each other face to face. I couldn't fathom the depth of my love, and I had no context for the depth of my fear.

The hospital buzzed with genteel nurses eager to help me to the bathroom and ensure Ryan's vitality. I didn't want to be discharged. I pleaded for Nurse Beth to secure Ryan into the car seat carrier so I knew he was safe, but she wouldn't do it. She needed to see that I could do it. I wished his fragile arm were protected in a baby sling. I was terrified of touching or moving it in such a way that the immobility would become permanent. In fact, I was scared of everything. Our wheelchair promenade to the car wasn't the jubilant jaunt I had envisioned. Twice, I asked the orderly to slow down. My heart swelled, but not with carefree pride or a peaceful sense of new beginnings. My chest was tight with unfamiliar responsibility and a new identity as Ryan's principal protector and provider. I repeated a silent prayer: Please let him live to experience his homecoming.

Halfway home, I made Doug pull over so I could sit in the back with Ryan. He wasn't crying, but the neck support insert I'd purchased for the car seat carrier didn't work, and his head flopped around if I didn't hold it upright.

Our transfer home was on a Saturday in October, so college football was a high priority for some. Doug offered frequent help from the couch while Ryan slept, and I fed the cat, retrieved the mail, and emptied the dishwasher, my regular routine after a couple of days away. I eventually squirreled away with Ryan to the nursery, which I had decorated to inspire tranquility, a nest of blue hues, velvety chenille, and enchanted woodland animals. It was time to live out my daydreams of endless cuddles and cozy kisses. Riding a wave of adrenaline, I pushed myself physically to unpack the hospital bags while Ryan slept in the bassinet. My body hurt. It felt like a bomb had gone off down there, and it was hard to stand up straight, like the musculature in my torso had turned to jelly. But it was my policy to unpack as soon as I returned from any trip. I looked over at Ryan at least every minute in adoration. And to be sure he was breathing. He was finally here, and I really had found the most adorable go-home outfit—the "nest effect" held for exactly 15 minutes until he started to stir.

The notebook with our feeding, sleeping, and diapering schedule was out and open, awaiting its first post-hospital entry. We were right on time. I knew Ryan would cry, and logic told me that one of a couple solutions would stop the crying. Let's solve this problem! As I'd been trained, I first checked his diaper. Great that it was dry, but was he dehydrated? Maybe he wasn't getting enough colostrum/early milk while we waited for the true inventory to arrive. My next move was to fill his belly, so I started the process of nursing him. And it *was* a process. It was nothing at all like the conversant mothers I'd seen nonchalantly offering a perfectly draped breast toward Baby's immediate satiation.

I got situated in the glider atop the inflatable innertube, unlatched my nursing tank, and let the udders hang loose. Little dignity remained following our birthing experience. I laid Ryan across the nursing pillow with his bad shoulder up, just as the lactation consultant had shown me, but he wasn't catching my nipple. We'd had success at the hospital just two hours prior. What was different? What was I doing wrong? Mental struggle shifted to physical pain, as one of the spools worth of stitches poked me like a thousand porcupines in my pants. I squirmed, trying to find a weight distribution that didn't annihilate my fourth-degree episiotomy or displace the gargantuan sanitary pad. I delicately switched Ryan to the other side, and he did latch but released way too quickly. I tried to shimmy my nipple into his little fish mouth, but his jaw wouldn't open wide enough. Without a latch, there would be no letdown. Thanks to the literature, I knew exactly what *wasn't* happening. The more upset Ryan became over the absence of farm-fresh milk, the less I could focus on proper technique and the more pressure I imposed. I couldn't feed my baby! I wasn't doing the only job I was charged with in the moment.

Over the ref's whistles, Doug heard Ryan's growing agitation and came to check on us. I sat up straighter and wiped the perspiration from my forehead.

"How we doin'?" he asked, staring at my exposed chest, a departure from my typically modest self.

"Fine, good," my voice quivered, but held, over Ryan's cries. "There are ups and downs, but we'll figure it out."

"I'm right out here if you need me," he said and walked out.

He didn't need to know. Back to figuring out how to feed our son.

And then I remembered. I had a couple single-serving bottles of formula I'd smuggled from the hospital. Research told me that supplementing with formula this early would be detrimental to my milk supply, but without thinking, I hooked Ryan up with the contraband. It was a quick fix, and the sweet sound of his suckling settled my nerves instantly. He downed the entire thing, burped with gusto, and fell right back asleep. I buried the bottle under some tissues in the waste basket and put Ryan back in the bassinet while I pumped to correct my (perceived) wrong. I'd review the nursing books and be ready for success at the next feeding.

In our first weeks together, I garnered the expertise of two different lactation consultants and pumped after every feeding, no matter what. Doug supported whatever I wanted to do, unfazed by the madness of nipple shields and a tube of formula taped to my breast. Feeding Ryan was squarely my department. Each feeding (up to 10 a day) was a decision to be grappled with, a decision I had to live with. How and what would I feed him?

He wailed through every attempted nursing session, while every bottle feeding was a breeze. The bottle really was the perfect paraphernalia, my ticket to success. While arduous, at least pumping eliminated a negative emotional exchange between me and my most important customer. The mechanical extraction and delivery of homemade nutrients via manufactured apparatus brought both of us temporary peace. On the contrary, each bottle of formula caused me much consternation and felt like a covert crime, in direct conflict with the "breast is best" billboards. But my body needed a break. I hadn't admitted to Doug that I was supplementing with formula as much as I was. My secret gnawed at me.

Doug was back to work quickly; paternity leave wasn't a thing back then. His life continued despite the small detail of having a wife and baby at home. He was gone from 8 am to 6 pm every day, and sometimes that was extended by a stop at the gym or drinks with coworkers. He always asked, but I wasn't good at saying no. He wasn't getting too much from me at that point, so the least I could do was to not be a ball-and-chain. I was the one with maternity leave, a break. I was the mother, and Ryan was my responsibility. By the time Doug got home, I had either tended to or hidden laundry piles, a tornado of bottles, strewn diapers, half-written thank-you cards, tear-filled tissues . . . the day's messes. I began to look the way I felt, exhausted and frazzled, but I managed to at least get my contacts in, ditch my robe by 4 pm, and slap a smile on my face—the happy mother. Dinner was on the table by 6:30 pm. Did Doug recognize his bride? Did he see the dark circles under my eyes and notice my waning ability to participate in intelligent conversation? What did he think? *Did* he think about it?

Ryan's firm preference to sleep in someone's arms contributed to my rudderless state. As deeply asleep as he might have appeared, he would awaken (and not quietly) like clockwork within 10 minutes of being placed in the bassinet or crib. I tried everything to stay in compliance with the sleep authorities' recommendations that Baby sleep in appropriate and stationary quarters. Sleep in motion—in the car, in a stroller, in a swing—was said not to count as true sleep. I even put a very low-power heating pad under the sheet to mimic human warmth and love, and I massaged him with lavender lotion to relax his nervous system. Ryan couldn't be tricked. I held him 18 to 20 hours a day, resulting in a certain loss of myself. My existence and purpose had shifted to sustaining his survival ahead of my own well-being. While blatantly irresponsible according to contemporary childcare standards, I slipped into the practice of lying down with him in my bed for his afternoon nap. The law is the law. But I also knew that for all of time and in regions of the world where cribs aren't an available asset, womankind has slept with her offspring. The main danger, I understood, was my suffocating Ryan. Even so, my sleep-deprived delirium convinced me that neither of us would let that happen, and my body's desperate need for sleep won out. I slept, but I sure didn't feel good about it. I didn't feel good about much. I kept trying to do what the books said, and I kept failing.

Ryan began projectile vomiting at least once out of every three feedings. His possessed body scared me every time, like a scene from *The Exorcist*. Were fast-flow bottle nipples the cause? Perhaps the bottles featuring gas-reduction technology would help? Would he be doing this if he were drinking from my breasts? How long did I need to hold him at a 45-degree angle after feeding to ensure it wouldn't come back up? The pediatrician wasn't concerned, which didn't quell my own concern. How could I know how much he was truly taking in when I couldn't measure what was ejected? Should I feed him more right away in order to check off a "full feeding," or wait the standard one and a half to two hours to feed him again? My mind spun constantly.

I accepted every request for visitors, imagining a distraction, an escape from my cycling thoughts. At least I wouldn't be alone if Ryan freaked out and would have someone to problem solve with. Chats about current events and my callers' lives would be a gateway to the world I once knew. Opening my door to guests was also a good reason to stay on top of personal hygiene and to keep smiling.

"Isn't it just pure bliss?" asked Aunt Margaret. "The best thing that's ever happened to you?" She seemed serious.

No, it felt more like torment. Was I the only one who thought so?

"It's the best and most important job you'll ever have," Mary proclaimed. "Congratulations on your promotion to CMO (Chief Mom Officer)!"

Well, if that were the case, it was depressing. Not only because I wasn't doing a good job but also because I didn't really like the job.

"Don't worry about a schedule in the early weeks. Just nurse him and hold him," Angela said. "It's whatever he wants; he's in charge."

Insanity! I couldn't just live my days in reaction to a 10-pound being. I needed some predictability, some order.

Instead of grounding conversations and stories of similar experiences, the visits shined a light on the euphoria of every other mother I knew. How natural caring for a brand-new human was to them, and how rewarding they found it all to be. I didn't mention that I fantasized about my other job, where I regularly received positive feedback. Instead, I feigned the ecstatic new mother and smiled outwardly. Inside, I felt like a dying fish being carried away by the current. I wasn't quite dead, but I no longer had any muscle or mental strength to swim. The conversations placed more tallies in the column of my failure, leaving me feeling even more alone and more fearful that I was doing it all wrong. I had been given this gift from the Universe and my father, and I couldn't enjoy it. Ryan deserved better.

    Fall has always been my favorite season, yet I hadn't been outside in days. I hadn't indulged in apple spice donuts, and I certainly hadn't spun up my usual gourd and mum display on the front steps. I had to pull my sh*t together. I missed having attainable daily goals. I missed using my brain in rational and creative ways. I missed my planner. Order and structure would help. I resolved to establish daily goals for us. They didn't need to be colossal; I would start small. Phase I: 9 am bath, 10 am tummy time with classical music for brain development ahead of feeding and a book at naptime before pumping. Thank you notes while he slept. Maybe a short walk before dinner. Phase II would be expeditions like bringing Ryan to the grocery store or Starbucks by myself. Baby steps.

    The sun, the crispest of blue skies, and the painted leaves called to me ever so quietly, reminding me that I was missing out. I decided to begin with a short walk around a couple of city blocks. If I kept to the circuit, we would never be more than five minutes from home. It wouldn't even require packing the diaper bag, and if he were to cry, the open air would absorb the noise. We wouldn't be disturbing too many for too long. It felt like a tangible, achievable, low-risk goal.

    Ryan was fed, diapered, and outfitted for the cooler temperatures. He waited contently in the swing while I pumped. Conscious of the ticking clock until he would again beckon for a bottle, I pulled on a pair of leggings fit for the outside world. I didn't bother with a bra and pulled a favorite hoodie over my sagging physique. I packaged Ryan in the fleece-lined carrier and clung to motivation and determination. We were going to do this; we were going to be like normal mothers and babies, enjoying a beautiful day, absorbing a little Vitamin D, and appreciating the splendor of new life.

I lugged the stroller down the front steps of our three-flat. Going for a walk had gotten complicated. Living in the city, we couldn't leave the stroller out, or it would be picked off. Ignoring a pang of hunger, I walked back inside and reached for the carrier. The stench was unmistakable. I unzipped the fleece, unfastened the five-point harness I'd finally mastered, and cautiously picked him up. I felt it immediately. The explosion went all the way up his back. He must not have noticed yet because he was still quiet.

It was no quick fix. Trying to stay positive and drawing on my nimble response to professional mishaps, I simply reassigned my daily goal. Instead of a walk, we'd have a bath. The walk could be tomorrow's goal. As I held him on my shoulder, another eruption, this time from the other end. What seemed like the entire contents of his last feeding shot across the room decorating the dining room rug. The silence broke, and we broke. We both wailed. My heart sank, and all remaining positivity faded. Screw the stroller. Let someone take it. We wouldn't be leaving the house before Ryan outgrew it anyway.

My knees weakened, and we slid slowly down the wall to the floor. In through the still open door blew a few leaves. Three stuck to my soaked sleeve like fly paper, adding to the swamp scene. My stomach turned. Fortunately, it was empty, or I would have retched just like Ryan. As if from outside my body, I observed the disaster, feeling the horror of it all. In that putrid moment, I knew what needed to happen. I would be better off back at the office, and Ryan would be better off being taken care of by someone who knew what she was doing. He deserved that much. Within minutes, I'd called the nanny agency I'd chosen from the dozens I'd queried. Through massive sobs, mine and Ryan's, my fingers navigated the phone as if they were sending the biggest and brightest SOS flare. Who went back to work early from maternity leave? I was a monster.

I heard the back door close. Doug was home early following an on-site client meeting. Unable to quickly collect myself, I was caught.

"Sarah, what in the . . ." he asked. "I won't ask what's wrong with Ryan, but what's wrong with you?"

"I can't do this," I said. "Every day is the same: Ryan cries, I change his diaper, feed him, pump, he throws up, I clean him up, hold him, and watch the clock until the next cry."

"Here, let me clean him up. You go shower and lie down," Doug offered, bending over to rescue Ryan. If he was horrified, he hid it well.

"I get nothing done, and neither of us is happy," I continued. "This is supposed to be the most joyous time of my life."

Defensive and ashamed, I handed Ryan over, managed to pull myself up, and walked out of the room without another word.

The shower stall enveloped me in steamy warmth and the prospect of cleanliness, washing away the morning. It was like the gentlest of bear hugs as the water ran down my back. Turning for shampoo, I winced as streams of water hit my nipples. I instinctively cupped them with my hands and stood in a protective pose, my face fully submerged beneath the showerhead. The tears weren't about the still-throbbing wounds between my legs or my stretchmark-streaked hips. Rather, indications were that I was failing at this new job. Drug-free, peaceful, and empowered births resulted in well-adjusted babies; Ryan endured a traumatic delivery and had cried a lot ever since. Babies learned facial expressions from their mothers; I rarely smiled. Socializing an infant was important; we didn't leave the house. Nursing promoted bonding; nursing wasn't working for us.

I sucked at this whole mothering thing. Was this a mistake? Like the biggest mistake of my freaking life? I used to have a life. Now I didn't, and Ryan was stuck with an unqualified person as his mother.

Feeling slightly more human with clean hair and clothes but unable to rest, I walked into the family room where Doug had Ryan on the playmat and was smiling and oohing and aahing at him. I wished I could do the same and mean it, actually have fun with my baby.

"Thanks," I said, sitting down next to the mat and rubbing Ryan's head.

"For what? I'm the kid's father," he said. "It's my job to help him . . . and you. Just tell me what to do, and I'll do it."

"That's the problem, Doug," I said, feeling agitated again. "I don't *know* what to do."

"What do you mean you don't know what to do?" he asked.

"Honestly, I don't even know what I mean or what the problem is," I said. "Maybe come with me to our pediatrician appointment tomorrow. I think we should talk to Dr. Tate. This just can't be right, any of it. Or maybe I should talk to my OB. I don't know."

"Let's start with Dr. Tate," Doug said. "I'm in."

My list of questions for her was on the long side but not egregiously so. I didn't want to be *that* patient. Sitting in the waiting room, I let my mind wander to my many prenatal appointments. I eagerly anticipated and enjoyed every visit. Who wouldn't? All eyes were on me—in a good way—especially as I blossomed in the third trimester. Literally all eyes: those of other expectant and hopefully expectant mothers and their significant others in the waiting room, sometimes a young child pointing with concerned curiosity, the doting nurses strolling and stationed in the corridors, and eventually the doctor. "You're absolutely glowing." "How are you feeling?" "You make it look easy." It was hard to leave that office without feeling like a superstar. It was approximately 45 minutes of the day fully dedicated to me. People asked about my well-being, monitoring all sorts of things to confirm that I was great. Perfect in one way (baby's heart rate), flawless in another (belly measurement), impeccable in yet another (my blood pressure). Ultrasound visits took the comfort and confidence to the next level. If Baby looked good, that meant I was performing well. Consistent with performance evaluations at work, I passed with flying colors. I was growing my baby well! There was never any doubt; the feedback was always positive.

Pediatrician visits were different. I hadn't mastered motherhood the way I had mastered pregnancy. What if the conclusion was, in fact, that I was a bad mom? Then what?

"Ryan," called the bubbly nurse in the doorway. I wondered if she had any choice but to be happy wearing pale yellow scrubs adorned with teddy bears.

"Yes, here," I said, still getting used to hearing his name called in place of mine. We were no longer one. He was the patient; the attention was now his, not mine. Kind of like going to the dog park, where everyone asks what your dog's name is but never yours.

"So, tell me. How's it going?" Betsy, the nurse, asked as we settled into the exam room with the hippopotamus exam table and jungle mural.

"It's amazing," I replied with a coy smile and a shoulder shrug. "Everything's going really well. Ryan is such a good baby, and we just love him so much."

What an idiot. Of course, we love our baby, and what do I have to prove to Bubbly Betsy anyway? Doug knew better than to alienate me with any modification to my statement. He smiled and nodded.

"Ryan looks great. I've got his measurements, and Dr. Tate will be in shortly," Betsy said.

It's a good thing we didn't have to wait long for Dr. Tate, or I might have lost my courage.

"Hi, team," Dr. Tate greeted us. Doug wore a Bears hat and had dressed Ryan in a Payton jersey.

"How is everyone?" she asked.

She searched for my eyes, which she had to wait for as they rose nervously from the floor. "How are YOU, Sarah?"

I wondered who'd tipped her off. From the time I'd interviewed Dr. Tate and the other pediatricians, I felt comfortable with her. She felt more like a friend than a medical professional. Still, until now, I hadn't needed to confide anything serious to her.

"Mmmm," I moaned, choking on the lump in my throat.

She came closer, placed a hand on my shoulder, and gave a gentle squeeze. "Take your time, Sarah. I want to hear this."

"I, I can't believe I'm saying this. But I have to, for Ryan," I managed. "We need... I think we need help."

I caught her making eye contact with Doug, whose pursed lips and nod confirmed the situation.

"Good," she said. "I know that was hard. It's hard to say it, and taking care of a baby *is* hard."

"Am I supposed to talk to you, or Dr. Roth?" I asked, ready to get the conversation over with.

"You're here, so tell me more," she said. "We're all here for you."

"I don't know where to start. Do you think he's fussy and doesn't sleep independently because of the bad delivery? I've read about how the circumstances of a baby's arrival can affect his temperament and chances in life," I asked but didn't give her a chance to respond. "It's really embarrassing to say, but I don't think I'm doing this right. Nothing I do makes him happy."

"Please don't be embarrassed," she said. "Actually, I wish more women would talk about this."

I put it all out there for Dr. Tate; it was the first Doug had heard much of it. The look on his face was mildly surprised, moderately concerned, and deeply supportive and loyal to me. I explained the circus of our feeding and pumping routine. I confessed to having given up nearly half of my self-prescribed pumping sessions, resulting in Ryan drinking more formula than expressed breast milk. More of the swamp water than the golden nectar. Saying it aloud exacerbated my selfishness and incompetence. To my surprise, Dr. Tate took a different angle and emphasized the importance of taking care of myself.

"Feeding a baby is a beautiful, life-sustaining act," she went on. "My wish for you is that you find a way of feeding Ryan that works—and is enjoyable—for *both* of you. Feeding him ought to be a sweet time, a time for him to receive sustenance from you, who loves him best."

I was hardly following and didn't know how to respond.

"Ryan has gotten six weeks of your milk and the associated immunities and pure love it represents," she went on. "Today's infant formula choices provide excellent nutrition and represent what I can see as an opportunity for you and Ryan to simplify things and enjoy each other more."

I paused at the new perspective. Was she giving me permission to let go of the feeding follies and feed him a diet of formula only? I wasn't ready to commit to abandoning him like that, but I did commit to considering it.

After I bared my soul, Dr. Tate examined Ryan, told us he looked perfect, and instructed me to make an appointment with Dr. Roth. She also firmly suggested I sign up for the "Transitions to Motherhood" group at Northwestern, the hospital where I'd delivered.

"It's a four-week seminar that's less of a class and more of a discussion group," she explained. "It's for new moms just like you who are looking to connect with other new mommies. They cover things like feeding and sleep, fussy babies, infant development, how your new addition impacts your marriage, and postpartum emotions."

Maybe she didn't understand. I *wasn't* interested in connecting. I just wanted to feel better. I wanted to like being a mother, and I wanted to be good at being a mother. I didn't need to be award-winning, but a step or two up from failing miserably would have been nice. I had only ever been to one group therapy session, and I really wasn't interested in another.

"Okay," I mumbled.

"So, you'll sign up?" she asked.

"She will. I'll be sure of it," Doug chimed in.

Apparently, I needed to be managed by Doug now.

I registered that night before he could bug me about it. There was one spot left, and the session started later that week. Serendipity, or another horrible decision? It would be my first car trip alone with Ryan. We bought the Volvo based on safety ratings, but no test dummy stats could diminish my anxiety about driving alone with him. While I wasn't worried about forfeiting the $60 I'd paid online, I knew I'd feel guilty not showing up and taking the spot from someone else.

Doug hung around much later than usual the morning of the group session. He stayed out of our way for the most part and didn't act like he was supervising. I knew, and he knew that I knew. He took Ryan to the other room while I got dressed in what I'd laid out the night before (but hadn't tried on). The aspirational low-rise, non-maternity corduroys and a thin sweater didn't quite work out. I improvised with velour lounge pants (a step up from leggings) and a cute chunky sweater. I made the biggest fuss over my hair since Ryan's arrival, and it felt good to make myself presentable. I should specify—presentable by my new standards. I wouldn't have been caught dead at the office like that. I remembered at the last minute to add disposable nursing pads to my bra. Disaster averted.

Turns out I surprised myself and didn't linger with the decision to stop pumping. I pumped for the last time the day after seeing Dr. Tate; it was nothing ceremonious. Circumventing my guilt, my psyche led me to make a clean break. I aspired to shift our feeding experience to a more positive one. I likened it to a tweak to the many strategic growth plans I'd worked on for clients.

The three of us walked out the back door together in silence, as if it were a typical exit. I felt like I was reporting to morning detention, although, of course, I'd never received a detention. Doug knew cheerleading wouldn't help. He snapped Ryan's carrier into the car, kissed me goodbye, and waited to get in his car until I pulled out of the garage. His surveillance was less than stealthy.

I told myself not to think about driving and to just do it, kind of like going to the gym. If I'd let myself think, I would've turned right around. My heart beat hard, and my white knuckles pulsed as I drove in the right-hand lane and Ryan cried. I didn't think. I didn't feel. I drove.

Fortunately, Ryan fell asleep five minutes ahead of our arrival, allowing me to find parking in peace and preventing the embarrassment of walking in with a shrieking baby. Beginning the night before, I'd reviewed the contents of the diaper bag more times than could be considered sane. For our two-hour outing, I had three bottles, five diapers, two changes of clothing, burp clothes, paper towel and cleaning supplies (in case he vomited), and six pacifiers. It was a big bag. As I shoved it into the mesh basket beneath the stroller, I realized I didn't have my purse. It was still in the kitchen. I could see it, placed perfectly on the counter, so I wouldn't forget it. I could have headed home with the legit excuse of not being able to pay the meter, but I pressed on. Still not thinking or feeling, we proceeded to the meeting room.

There was a first day of school feeling in the air. Two of the babies slept, and their mothers were seated. Most of the ladies kinetically swayed or bounced in the hopes of keeping their precious bundles quiet. We went around the table with introductions as a couple of late arrivals settled in. Everyone was a first-time mother, so either still on maternity leave or climbing the new ranks of stay-at-home motherhood. The first monologues were as expected: thick with the superfluous joys of motherhood, all rosy depictions. This was the same BS I'd heard before. Then something surprising happened. A woman named Etta admitted she hadn't slept for more than two hours a day in five weeks and was close to cracking. Brie said she felt like a single parent even though she was married. Rebecca's baby, Marty, cried non-stop with no diagnosis and therefore no solution, which, in turn, made her cry. Her swollen face confirmed as much. Lindy couldn't let go of deep disappointment about her C-section. Nila didn't know how to nicely tell her mother-in-law that she didn't want her around. Once the seal was broken, a candid cascade commenced, and one admission was followed by another was followed by another.

These women didn't look like failures to me. They looked like women who had temporarily lost their luster in trying really, really hard. Trying so hard to acclimate to a startling, new existence where someone else always came first. Trying to bear the incredible weight of incremental and ultimate responsibility. Trying to remember who they once were. Trying to understand who they were now. I hadn't expected the raw reveals. It was as if the exhaustion had stripped the women of their inhibitions. Another surprising something happened.

"I'm Sarah, and this is Ryan," I said. "This might sound a little strange, but does anyone else ever feel . . . kind of scared? Scared to be home alone with your baby?"

"Totally," Laura said. "I start getting scared around sunset. I'm terrified of the nights. They're so long. I've started leaving all the lights on all the time."

Brie chimed in, "I asked my mom to stay on speaker phone once for hours just so I wasn't alone as Matty screamed his heart out."

I wasn't the only one!

"Ah, I feel so much better," I said, nearly out of breath with relief. "I've been so freaked out lately that I called the nanny agency the other day, weeks before I actually need to go back to work."

"What do you mean? Why did you call?" someone asked.

"I guess because I don't feel like I'm doing a good enough job for Ryan," I said almost under my breath, chin low and instantly regretful. "The thought of someone who knows what they're doing taking care of Ryan and my returning to work, where I know what I'm doing, felt like a light at the end of the tunnel."

"Sarah! Oh, my goodness, get the help," Brie said. "I mean, if you can swing it, can you bring in the nanny a little early? Just get some help?"

"I don't know," I said. "The help would be great since my mom isn't retired yet and my mother-in-law is busy. But I'm supposed to be able to take care of my own kid."

"Totally, what Brie said," Nila added. "You don't need to deserve it; there's no shame in getting help. I don't know what I'd do without my mom's weekly help, and it sounds like you don't have that kind of hands-on support. I actually don't think anyone is meant to mother alone."

"You can have my mother-in-law, if you'd like," she threw in with a giggle.

It was better than misery loving company. It was group coaching! Just like Dr. Tate's idea to give up pumping, I had to marinate on the grandiose idea of getting help. I wasn't ready to talk to Doug about it. What would he think? It wasn't in the budget. Anyway, the work was mine, and I had to figure it out. Yet, I did feel the slightest twinge of hope at the prospect.

Showing up at class that first day was the hard part. The barrier to sharing the truth and asking for help was lowered from there. Over the course of the next three weeks, I opened up more and more. We all did. We learned to be vulnerable, first by observing and then by finding the courage to speak our own truths. We laughed, and we cried. Realizing that we weren't the only ones thinking and feeling what we had made us giddy. I'd harbored so much shame in doing things "against the books" instead of embracing that I was doing what I had to do to survive. What worked for me and Ryan was what made me the best mother I could be. These ladies were a counter resource to the books, a living, breathing human resource. Most of us were the first among our friends to have children. While steadfast, loyal, and long-term, our existing friendships didn't offer intrinsic support for our new, uncharted circumstances. We found lifelines in each other, and almost like a new romance, we couldn't get enough.

We met up outside of class and did normal mom and baby things like go to the park, shop for baby clothes we definitely didn't need, and organize playdates. There might have even been a glass of something involved if it was after 3 pm. I went into their homes, saw their messes, and showed them mine. No one cared. Together, we even dared to eat at restaurants. If someone's baby cried, we all jumped to help. We analyzed the trite and the profound—everything from which cocoa butter was best for stretch marks and which diapers didn't leak to our thinning hair and first postpartum intimacies. All the things non-mothers didn't care to discuss but around which our days revolved. My world opened up.

In addition to the group dynamic, Brie and I hit it off immediately and texted and talked directly with increasing frequency. Each time we talked, often in the evening while our hubbies were still at work or traveling, we determined another synchronicity in our lives. One of the biggest gifts of truth we exchanged early on was around how many children each of us desired.

"I know for sure I'm having only one child, and I told Doug as much the other night," I said. "We have so much we want to do, like travel."

"That's us," Brie laughed. "I totally agree that one is plenty. One and done!"

I'm not sure what astonished me more: the ladies' encouragement to get help or the fact that I listened to them. They pointed out all the evidence that I wasn't failing (Ryan was still alive, he was growing, he was dressed), and they led us to Kenzie, my beautiful partner in loving and caring for Ryan. Something in me shifted after hiring her. She helped us half-days two days a week until I went back to work. As I onboarded her and familiarized her with our routines, I realized how far Ryan and I had come. I did know a few things after all. We did a lot with him together, co-mothered, so he didn't feel passed off. I probably didn't want to feel so quickly replaceable either. Knowing he was cared for, I also took the opportunity to indulge in things like untimed showers, meetups with old friends, and some light exercise since my body was again mine. It's amazing what can be accomplished in just a few hours a week. My head and heart calmed and merged in a way they hadn't before coexisted.

I gained beautiful perspective in my three remaining weeks at home with Ryan. I registered the miraculous amongst the hard and scary. When he started smiling for real (about more than gassies), it was an answer to my need for feedback. Through his smiles and in his eyes, my native love grew to new dimensions. I was able to take in the moments I would pay so much to be able to revisit today: the uniquely marvelous softness at the base of his neck, my favorite place to bury my nose; the sweet, sweet sound of his suckling on the nipple (flesh or silicone, it didn't matter); his fingers around mine or reaching for my face. As he started to adapt to sleeping somewhere other than my arms, I would still check every 15 minutes to be sure he was breathing. Even so, I was starting to feel worthy of my new best friend even if I wasn't perfect. My newfound support changed everything for me and made my transition back to work as smooth as it could be. I eventually struck a healthy balance, and I had the best of both worlds.

Late that first summer, I had an idea. I needed to share it with Doug since the idea's execution would require his participation. The three of us walked around Lincoln Park one beautiful Saturday afternoon, which felt like the perfect opportunity to throw out a lofty topic without sitting across from Doug and looking him in the eyes.

"I've been thinking," I said.

"Uh, oh. What's up?" Doug asked.

"Well, it might make sense to have a second soon."

"A second what?" he asked.

"Second child," I responded, aware of the shock value of what was rolling off my tongue.

"Hon, I think you're a little delirious right now," he said. "Maybe you're still buzzed from that second glass of wine last night. You've made it extremely clear that you want only one child."

"When things were so hard with Ry, I told myself one was enough," I chuckled nervously. This was an important sale I was trying to make. "But now I'm thinking it makes sense to just knock it out, be in crazyville for a couple years straight, and be done with it."

"Please don't go into planning mode right now. Can we just enjoy Ryan and everything we have going for us?" he proposed. "What's meant to be will find its way to us in due time."

I agreed with the concept, but my need for a firm plan was insatiable. "Due time" didn't do it for me. In a follow-up conversation, Doug reminded himself that as an only child, he'd always wanted his own children to have a sibling or more. We agreed to let whatever might happen, happen. I was leaving for an annual business conference a few days later and wanted to say a nice good-bye. So, we did just that. Given that the meeting was in San Antonio that year, I forwent the margaritas at our client event just in case. Sure enough, Michael took root along the River Walk and joined us 20 months after Ryan's blessed, albeit messy, arrival.

Chicago's Northern Suburbs, Many Years Later

Dearest Ryan,

I thought I was ready; I really did. How humbling to then find caring for you to be so foreign, scary, and confusing. God gifted you to me, entrusted you to me. You, in turn, bestowed on me a litany of gifts: trust, grace, courage, grit, and honesty, to name a few. Thank you for your patience as I integrated into motherhood, stretched into my new job. I'm sure you could sense my unsteadiness, and I pray that on some level you've always known that you could count on me.

Thank you, too, for leading me to the new motherhood group. My need to care for you by way of caring for myself brought me to my fellow vulnerable mothers. I was rewarded for telling the truth. I was freed, and then I was myself reborn into the mother, wife, friend, and human I have become and continue to evolve to be. Those ladies became my tribe. Their embrace, their honesty, and their love fueled me. This I know: I will forever be better for having been your mother.

With so much love,
Your Mama

Chapter 2

Fab Four

DANIELLE

*"You are braver than you believe,
stronger than you seem, and smarter than you think."*
—Christopher Robin, *Winnie the Pooh*

Scott and I took the morning off and turned the ultrasound appointment into a mini date. I even curled my hair. We dropped Claire off at daycare and grabbed breakfast at our favorite diner. I rationed my pancake, bacon, and decaf intake so I wouldn't be uncomfortable on the exam table. And just in case the wand happened to wander across any of my own organs, I didn't need any judgment of their contents. We had a great morning, and I did a decent job of curbing the nerves associated with the notorious 20-week anatomy scan. I focused on the opportunity to see Baby on the 4D technology and add the images to my mounting collection.

The energy in the waiting room was unsettling, the comingling of everyone's circumstances in being there. Many were presumably exultant, some sad, and others desperate. Scanning the magazine headlines and glossy brochures decorating the tables,

I reminded myself I had nothing to worry about. The office was running on-time for once, and we were called back before we had too much time to sit idle and perseverate. Still, a lump formed in my throat as we approached the ultrasound room.

"Before we get started, I want to confirm that you *do* want to know Baby's sex," said Sandy, the tech. She was nice enough but didn't emanate much warmth as she exposed my burgeoning belly and prepared to take the closest of looks.

"We already know we're having a boy," I explained, trying to get comfortable while at the same time evading the irritating crinkle of the table's paper lining. "Being 35 makes me geriatric in the obstetric community, so I had bloodwork done at 10 weeks. Everything was great, so no worries about spoiling any surprises!"

"And this is your second pregnancy," Sandy said. "Who do you have at home?"

"Our sweet Claire," I said. "Two years, heavy medication, too many injections, and five IUIs later, we got pregnant naturally, and she got comfy in that perfectly tilted uterus you see right there."

"Got it," she said. "Was it any easier this time around?"

"Actually, yes." I smiled, the lump in my throat dissipating as I recalled our smooth path to this pregnancy. "I had baby fever something fierce and went straight to the fertility clinic to get my Clomid. I was pregnant within three months. When I got the plus on the test stick, I was so shocked I wet my pants even though I'd relieved myself onto the stick just five minutes earlier. We're so lucky."

Sandy drew lines all over the big screen. I tried to keep up with her mouse clicks and really wanted to understand what we were looking at, but she didn't say much. Her job was to take meticulous measurements, not to provide color commentary, but an embellishment here or there would've been nice. I watched with increasing anxiety as she scrutinized his developing heart, brain, neck, spine, kidneys, bladder, arms, legs, hands, fingers, feet, toes, lips, chin, nose, eyes, face, chest, lungs, stomach, and intestines. I remembered from Claire that the appointment was long. But as my bladder inevitably filled, I was antsy to get dressed and go down the hall to Dr. Blakely's office for the debrief.

I love Dr. Blakely. She was with me through Claire's pregnancy and is someone I could see myself having cocktails with if she didn't so regularly have her eyes and hands in my hoo-hoo. I looked forward to my appointments because we always laughed, and I came to trust her implicitly with my health and that of my babies. I could ask her any question and talk about anything that was on my mind with no concern of judgment.

I remember exactly three good things about that scan: 1) The warm gel; 2) The magnificent topography of Baby's face; and 3) Scott's incredible support. The list of bad things was shorter than the list of good things. There was only one bad thing, but that one thing felt colossal on that day . . . and insurmountable for the days and weeks to come.

"Good morning, you two," Dr. Blakely said. "It's so great to see you both again."

"Hey, Doc," Scott responded, flexing his boy-dad muscles a bit. "Are you ready for this little dude? He can't possibly be cooler than Claire, but he'll be *as* cool."

"Oh, yes. I'm very ready," she said.

"Okay, tell us everything," I blurted. Enough with the small talk. I needed to hear that everything was okay.

"Most everything on the scan is as expected, and Baby is healthy," Dr. Blakely started. "However, he does have bilateral clubfoot or talipes equinovarus."

My jaw dropped slowly, and the blood drained from my face. She didn't have much of a choice but to give me a minute, or a few. My sobs echoed against the undecorated walls. I figured my second pregnancy would go as smoothly as the first, and so the blow hit high and hard. Dr. Blakely walked around from behind her desk, leaned in, and looked in my eyes with compassion and confidence.

"Danielle, everything else looks good so far," she said. "Clubfoot is common, and it's very treatable. I know it's hard to hear that something isn't exactly perfect with your baby, but this *is* going to be okay."

As my sobbing temporarily quieted, she explained a bit more about clubfoot and our next steps. We had earned the label and stigma of "high risk," not a designation any expectant mother covets. She offered for us to exit the office through the back door, a detour to avoid walking through the waiting room. In that kindness, she was granting me privacy, and she was also protecting those anxiously awaiting their own appointments and destinies. We were thrown onto the diagnostic path of weekly scans to determine any associated conditions or root causes of Baby's diagnosis. They looked for—and I lost sleep over—things like a hole in his heart or malformations of his spine. My melodic weeping continued and stopped only long enough to conduct work calls and to show up for two-and-a-half-year-old Claire as a person she recognized.

Clubfoot typically results from one of the following: a hereditary birth defect, an awkward fetal position in-utero, or an underlying co-condition such as Downs Syndrome, Spina Bifida, Arthrogryposis, or Dwarfism. The clinic's scanning protocol, along with the newly acquired knowledge that my father had clubfoot, gave the medical professionals—and us—the solace of our baby's clubfeet being hereditary and not a symptom of something bigger or worse. Everything else repeatedly checked out month after month, and we were finally released from further diagnostic imaging.

Even so, I wasn't celebrating. That winter, I wallowed over

our baby's future missed milestones and in not knowing how this would affect him, both in infancy and beyond. How different would he be? Would he need special shoes? Would he ever play soccer? Hockey? Rock climb? My persistent pondering ballooned into a state of general disheartenment. Google didn't help my spiraling mind, and we wouldn't know the severity of his deformity until birth. Basically, there are two types of clubfoot: positional clubfoot, which can be treated non-surgically via stretching, exercise, and massage, and fixed clubfoot, which requires more invasive treatment, including casting and surgery.

One evening after prepping and cleaning up dinner, Scott interrupted my regular couch-based blubbering with a proposition.

"Let's get the heck outta here and head to the beach," he said with more than natural enthusiasm. He bit the inside of his cheek and raised his eyebrows, anticipating my response. I admit I was a little volatile during that time.

"Mmmm," I responded. "I don't know. I don't know if I want to see people."

"Dani, we need to break this cycle," Scott said. "I'll do all the packing, and you don't need to talk to anyone but Claire and me if you don't want to."

"I don't know," I muttered. Even with Scott handling all the details, I didn't have the energy. I refocused my attention to my iPad.

"Okay, please really think about it," he pleaded. "I think it could be good for us, for all of us."

He didn't leave me much ground for refusal. By the next afternoon, Scott had put the plans in motion, including pulling my summer maternity clothes out of storage. How many guys dare to get involved with off-season clothing? He knew I wouldn't be caught dead at the beach in my then daily uniform of yoga pants and oversized t-shirt. I love resort wear and always had fun planning matching vacation dresses for me and Claire. He knew me so well.

Thank goodness for my ever reliable and thoughtful husband because that trip was my turning point. I can hardly explain it other than to describe that spending time with Scott and Claire in the sun and surf reset me. Just for the record, I did speak with a few select others, mostly those who could set me up with my craving of the day.

The reality of many unknowns continued, but a perspective found its way from the sand into my heart and mind. I consciously decided to take Dr. Blakley's word for it and set out to believe that it *was* going to be okay. Our beautiful boy had no other issues. We would deal with his feet the best we possibly could, and somehow, it *would* be alright. While I wish this perspective had come to me sooner, it came exactly when it needed to, and it placed us on an entirely new and brighter path.

As soon as we returned home to Nashville, I booked a pregnancy photo shoot. I also began extensively researching the right orthopedic practice to help us upon his arrival and settled on a group at Vanderbilt. Just having that plan helped tremendously. I educated myself, which empowered me against the daunting mystery of what his arrival might bring. Making and working a plan was what I did well, and it allowed me to embrace the remainder of my pregnancy and to anticipate his arrival with new hope and pleasure.

It was time to name him, and finding the perfect name took us longer than it did with Claire. We eventually narrowed the options to three and tried them all out—talking to each other and to him directly. The exercise brought his name to life, and we eventually landed on Benjamin, to be called Benny.

Throughout the remainder of my pregnancy and during my labor and delivery, I advocated for myself in ways I didn't know how to with Claire. I was emboldened with goddess energy as only a laboring mother is. I spoke up to postpone the epidural and asked for guidance with pushing positions. I didn't just lie there hooked up to monitors and IV lines waiting for "it" to happen. The entire experience was more positive and productive the second time around. Our Benny's safe arrival was followed by scrumptious snuggles, all the usual newborn assessments, and a few extra looks from the orthopedic squad. As it turned out, Benny had fixed clubfoot (the more severe variety), which had his feet turned very tightly inward. I must say, the entire situation didn't feel *as* freakish as I had originally imagined it would.

Sure, we had a challenge to deal with, but that's what Scott and I did so well together. We had weathered career bobbles, family drama, and many home-buying decisions. My sighs of relief were deep and therapeutic. We could do this. And I finally had a child who somewhat resembled me! I got lost in Benny's eyes, his dark hair, and his olive skin tone. Gorgeous Claire is a spitting image of Scott, which is funny considering the non-dominant traits that entails. But with Benny, even as a newborn, someone off the street would associate him with me, and that felt amazing. Those first hours together were magical.

Caring for Benny early on felt just like caring for any newborn, and I was more confident this time, many thanks to my guinea pig, Claire. His umbilical cord didn't make me queasy, holding him felt natural, and I wasn't ashamed of giving him a pacifier. It almost felt like I knew what I was doing. One consequence of his feet's formation was that he was prone to kicking himself during diaper changes. Fortunately, there was no damage done other than my sadness and helplessness. Lots of newborns wear those cute little mittens to cover sharp nails their parents are too scared to manicure, but there wasn't anything I could place on Benny to protect him from his own feet. At least not yet.

The honeymoon ended with Benny's one-week appointment with the orthopedic surgeon. Walking into the office felt very different from a routine visit to the pediatrician. We were there because there was something wrong with our baby. My heart pounded as I checked us in and until we were in the presence of Dr. Yun. I knew he was the right partner for us on this mission. We were expecting a consultation that day, but we walked out with both of Benny's little legs in casts. I'm grateful Dr. Yun was as clear and convincing as he was about getting started that day because the only positive thing to hold on to at that point was that the sooner we started, the sooner we would be finished.

Each week for two months, Benny had new casts put on to slowly turn his feet outward. Our color options were red, white, and blue, so we switched it up and planned fun outfits around his new fashion accessories. Turns out white leg casts aren't ideal for a baby, given their tendency to trap dirt and everything else that's brown. Benny's casts led to our family's imprisonment for the next two months. He screamed non-stop when he wasn't asleep. His inability to bend and stretch his legs meant he couldn't pass gas effectively. We massaged his belly and held him in all the indicated positions, but we couldn't pump his legs the way we did for Claire. He was miserable and in turn, so were we. We couldn't take him anywhere, and Claire's narrative to anyone who would listen was always, "Benny cries." Nothing about his toys or books, nothing about his glorious scent (most of the time) and nothing about his delicious thigh rolls. From the mouths of babes. It was true—Benny cried. That's how I remember it because that's how it was.

His continuous shrieking, coupled with the physicality of two heavy casts, made our magical mommy-baby moments far and few. There were no dramatic readings of *Goodnight Moon*, no singing lullabies, and no gazing lovingly into each other's eyes.

"Dani. Danielle. DANIELLE," Scott beckoned upon returning from the park with Claire one fall afternoon. "Hon, where are you?"

"What?" I asked, snapping back to consciousness.

"It's like you're not here," he said. "Benny's crying. Why aren't you doing anything?"

"Nothing I do helps," I said. "He just ate and burped. His diaper's clean. I tried rocking him. I walked him around the block. Nothing works, so now I'm just trying to ignore it."

Scott saw it on my face; I didn't want to hold Benny. I was empty. There was nothing there: no happiness, no sadness, no rage. Nothing. Postpartum depression was not something on our radar. I didn't have issues with Claire, just the typical psychosis around SIDS and a broad set of fears including but not limited to failure to thrive, drowning in the bath, or breaking her arm wrangling her into a sleeper. I was always scared and always wondered if she was okay, but it seemed to be on the scale of normal. As I think back, the lack of connection I felt with Benny was terrifying. Scott calculated it more than I did, but I recognized it on some level. I knew I wasn't supposed to be despondent about my precious child.

My initial bouts of panic had eased and were replaced by catatonia as my nerves sizzled and fried. I think my mental and physical selves morphed into some type of survival mode. Because I couldn't help Benny and because it was so very agonizing to my soul to hear his pain, I disconnected and shut down. It was not by any conscious act; it just happened. That's my own non-medical assessment. I'm sure there are chapters about the phenomenon in psychology textbooks and obstetrics journals.

Scott was confident he could support me through this time, and I wanted to believe it too. I promised Scott I was fine and that Benny and I would be fine. But things didn't get better right away. Scott's comment one day as he left for work is seared in my mind. "If you think you're going to hurt yourself or hurt the baby, please tell me."

My response did nothing to increase his confidence in leaving.

"I would never hurt my child, but I can understand why people might shake their babies."

Even with those worrisome words said out loud, we thought we could get through it on our own. We did, but I don't suggest anyone try the same at home. In hindsight, there is so much help available. We didn't need to suffer like that. At the time, I thought Scott was all I needed, and he *was* my number one supporter. He hurried home from work the day I called to announce that I couldn't do it anymore. Without parents who were local and/or available to support us on a daily basis, we had only each other, and I needed more of his help. We took turns with Benny so we wouldn't lose our minds and so we could both spend quality time with Claire. Those first two months blurred together, and each day was as difficult as the last. There was no reprieve from the crying, and there was no opportunity for a turnaround trip to the beach. Resort security would have had us escorted out. All in all, it was pretty terrible, but we got through it by leaning on each other, urgently awaiting Benny's release from the casts, and focusing on our hope for the future.

A different child was born when the last set of casts came off. Benny's crying stopped almost immediately, and he blossomed into the charismatic and sweet personality he is today. My psyche was subsequently restored, and Benny and I started anew with our relationship. It was like we were dating. We picked up where we had left off on day seven before the casts, and we bonded in all the natural ways, making the next phase of treatment infinitely more tolerable. He endured surgery to lengthen his tendons and was relegated to his "magic boots" post-op. The boots have a metal bar between them that keeps his feet in the proper position. Pinterest came through, and I found colorful fabric covers to put over the bars—anything to divert his (and my) attention from the device. Initially, he wore the boots for 23 hours a day, seven days a week. We had spa time during his single hour of daily freedom: a bath and a massage.

He missed out on a lot of skin-to-skin contact, being casted right away and then braced. After three months of 23/7 wear, we slowly phased him into nighttime boot wear only, which he's done for the past year and a half. He'll wear the boots at night until he's five years old, and I will continue to adorn the bar with my collection of cute coverings.

Our rocky start means I will never take our current closeness for granted. I carry heavy guilt about my early disconnection from Benny as a young baby who couldn't help his discomfort and boisterous expression of it. Sadly, the end of Benny's casting and surgical phase coincided with my return to work. Just as he had calmed and calibrated, and we had fallen deeply in love, I had to leave him. The return didn't bother me as much with Claire, but I had enjoyed that maternity leave. With Benny, I had an intense sense of making up for lost time; we had a ton of unfinished business between us. It infuriates me that in this country, women are forced to give up their babies to a stranger after only a few weeks . . . in order to work to live.

We finally found our rhythm not too long ago, and I'm feeling like myself again. From here, I can see that Benny's diagnosis wasn't the end of the world. Not even close! The time went fast. It was impossibly difficult at times. But. We. Did. It. Scott, Claire, Benny, and I did it together, and here we are, on the other side of it, looking forward to all that lies ahead for this extraordinary boy. In his strength and with his (loud) voice, he taught me how strong I am.

I was stronger because of Scott, too. He and I will always draw from those 33 weeks (the back half of my pregnancy plus the first three months of Benny's time here) and reflect on how we battled. We survived because we had a strong foundation going in and worked together, and that period is now further infrastructure for enduring life's twists and turns that are sure to come.

I'm super grateful that I've mandated bi-annual family photos even though they aren't always (okay, aren't ever) a popular activity. Despite any given day's storm, I also have first-year monthly milestone photos for both Claire and Benny. We didn't miss one. Today, when I see the early photos of Benny, his screams aren't my first remembrance. I smile at good memories, confirmation that every member of our family is indeed brave, strong, and smart.

If you use social media at all, you've likely caught onto the recent attention paid to "national days." Although some national days, like National Hot Dog Day and National Underwear Day seem silly to me, I will now always recognize National Clubfoot Day. Here is an excerpt from my post this year on the special day:

> If I could go back and tell my 20-week pregnant self anything, it would be to wipe away those tears. It's going to be okay. Benny is perfect and so strong. While this will always be a part of who he is, we will forever do all we can to support him so that no door is shut for him. The day Benny walks independently will be a day to celebrate! Along the way, we met a wonderful community of clubfoot parents and have been blessed with support from our wonderful orthopedic team at Vanderbilt. Clubfoot babies are born one in 1000, and we are beyond thankful for our clubfoot cutie.

Newsflash: Benny walked on his own at 13 months. There were no missed milestones after all. Go, Ben Ben! Go, Benny Boy! You are a champion, *our* champion!

I'd be lying by way of withholding information if I didn't share that there were moments I regretted my pregnancy with Benny. I beat myself up over that and am always working to forgive myself for what was likely a self-protection mechanism. And once he was here, it was a struggle. If

Benny had been our first child, I likely would have closed up that shop. We're humans, mere humans, and our individual thoughts at any given point in time don't define us. What defines us is how we sit with and assess those thoughts to inform our path forward.

Society dictates that women are made to do this, to become—and be instantly happy as—mothers. Our physical bodies are equipped to conceive, carry, and deliver babies. Yet, having a baby is not the same as being a mother. Our bodies are ready, but what other element of us is primed for the destabilizing transition? In fact, it really *isn't* a transition at all. My life went from being pretty composed to having someone screaming in my face most of every day. I was thrown to the wolves, or a single wolf. Becoming a mother is nothing short of a woman's own rebirth. We instantaneously take on a new identity, one in which we are to unconditionally love someone we've only just met. Coming to love someone is usually a process. Hence, the phrase "falling in love" and certain conditions or criteria foster and sustain that love. Not in the scenario of motherhood, though. We get no time to change costumes or to paint on our new faces for our new roles. We immediately and forever become someone new, someone different.

We need to talk more about this. We need to support each other throughout the entire process of becoming and being mothers, from fertility challenges and pregnancy concerns to delivery complications and postpartum depression. We need to discuss that love doesn't always happen immediately. We need to connect more about *everything*: the good, the bad, and the ugly. And I'll kick off the discussion by offering to you, dear reader, four resources that have gotten me through. They have been indispensable to my survival and my sanity.

My Fab Four are these:

1. **A solid partner.** If you happen to be reading this prior to selecting a mate/co-parent/spouse, please prioritize the characteristic of a 50-50 partner. Or, if you have made your selection and haven't yet had a child, please take the time to discuss *in advance* how you plan to divide and conquer and work together under any and all (including unforeseen) circumstances. It makes all the difference between the good days and the bad days. It makes the entire parenting experience better, more rewarding, and more awesome. Parenting *together* gets my vote. And if you're a single parent, that absolutely doesn't mean you have to be alone. Seek out and surround yourself with people to support you . . . they're out there just waiting to help!

2. **A fabulous OB/Gyn or midwife**, maybe even a doula. A neighbor recently shared her choice of a random OB from her insurance plan's roster. In an uncharacteristic rant of unsolicited commentary, I urged her to interview multiple providers and to choose carefully because this individual will be a key player on this turbulent (even if nothing goes wrong, per se) 9-month journey. I encourage you to please do the same. Do yourself and your baby the honor of finding a doctor or midwife who truly listens to you, with whom you can discuss anything, and who inspires your confidence in pregnancy, postpartum, and motherhood in general.

3. **Clinical emotional support**, if you think you might need it. There is no shame in having a hard time and not being able to pull out of a fog or funk. I know you're not making it up. And I know you're brave, strong, and smart. But passing through the powerful gates to motherhood transforms us forever, and that's a big deal. We aren't meant to weather the transformation alone. There is abundant help available, and your OB or pediatrician can guide you to it.

4. **Mighty mama buddies.** Nothing beats the support of those who understand firsthand, those who are living a version of your experience. They see you clearly because they *are* you. You might be lucky enough to have these ladies organically built into your life as a sister, sister-in-law, or friend. While those who have been mothers before us are helpful resources, there is something uniquely valuable in the camaraderie of going through an experience together, at the same time. At the very least, join one or more online communities. And ideally, find an in-person forum where everyone is vulnerable and can relate to what you're going through. Believing that we aren't alone is incredibly powerful medicine.

You've got this, Mama!

Chapter 3

Clueless with a Capital "C"

MONICA

> *"Shame cannot survive being spoken.*
> *It cannot tolerate having words wrapped around it.*
> *If we share our story with someone who responds*
> *with empathy and understanding, shame can't survive."*
> —Brené Brown

It was almost too easy. After settling into our marriage for two years, Jeff and I were ready to embark on parenthood. We had hit our respective career strides, prepared a modest starter home on the beautiful North Shore of Chicago, and indulged our wanderlust. I was on-track—or even a little ahead—with my five-year plan. I felt no qualms, only eager anticipation of motherhood, of what would be the best thing that ever happened to me. I knew change was coming, but I didn't focus on it. Contrary to my passionately planful self, I just kind of figured it would all work out. Having kids was what people did. I stopped taking my birth control pills and waited for my first period. "Trying" was relaxed and fun since we were ahead of the ticking clock. I held great promise for our new chapter together.

On Night 26 of my next cycle, I tossed and turned, my mind full and swirling. As I eventually laid wide awake in the wee hours, I held my bladder as long as I could. I wanted that first trip to the bathroom to be perfect: highly concentrated urine chock full of HCG (Human Chorionic Gonadotropin). How at-home tests work was about the extent of my knowledge of pregnancy; I did understand that much. Jeff knew I had purchased a box of tests, but I didn't tell him I had plans to use one. The test instruction I didn't heed was waiting until at least the first day of a missed period, and preferably a week after, for a more accurate result. I couldn't wait any longer. That's why they sell boxes of three tests, right? I could take another the next day and then the next. I peed on the end of the stick and replaced the cap. I couldn't stand watching it for three full minutes, so I took a quick shower and shaved my legs while the paper strip absorbed and processed my future.

The ecstasy of the second pink line was indescribable. I felt that line in my heart, in my head, and in every cell of my being. It wasn't even faint; it was bold and brilliant and beautiful. I was pregnant! There was no creativity in how I delivered the news to Jeff. No corny t-shirt, no new daddy cigar. I wasn't good with secrets and had to tell him immediately. I crawled back into the still-warm sheets and slipped my arm over his back and around his waist. Given our recent uptick in purposed intimacy, he reasonably assumed I was ready to go again. He turned over and began caressing me but immediately noticed my tears. I handed him the stick without words, and his tears quickly exceeded mine. How blessed we were, and we would not take it for granted.

We waited a bit to share our news, and the secret between us was electrifying. Knowing something so spectacular, just the two of us, drew us even closer. I saw my beloved OB/Gyn to confirm the pregnancy, and I was on top of the world. Four weeks passed quickly. We chose Washington Gardens, one of our favorite Italian eateries, for our official celebration, and that evening just felt different. While I didn't yet feel or look different physically, my identity began to shift. As Jeff held the car and restaurant doors for me, it hit me that he was doing so for me *plus one*. I felt special, maybe even the slightest bit royal.

Our waitress, Angie, was one we had come to know well. Upon asking if I'd like my regular glass of Cabernet, I sat up a little straighter, smiled and asked for a Cranberry and soda with a lime. While we had planned to tell family first, I blurted out, "I'm expecting!" Saying it aloud felt surreal. Caught off guard by my breach of plan but quickly back on his feet, Jeff chimed in to share how easily we'd become pregnant, our due date, and how we wanted to be surprised by the baby's gender. Angie's nods, smiles, and questions seemed genuine, like more than schmoozing for a good tip. She already knew we were good tippers. Listening to Jeff talk about our baby to someone else made it feel more real. That was the night I stepped into my new status as an expectant mother.

At some point midway through dinner, Brent caught my eye and came over to greet us. He was a friend from the neighborhood and a local radiologist. Perhaps because the seal on our secret had been broken, or perhaps as an explanation for the gigantic portion of chicken parmesan on my plate, I again reported our pregnancy. Brent quickly asked who my doctor was, and I told him how much I loved Dr. Kass.

"Monica," he said. "You know, when it comes to delivering babies, it's really more about the hospital than the doctor. Highland Park Hospital doesn't have a NICU."

He was clear in the directive to change doctors so I could deliver at Lutheran General, whose NICU is renowned. "I recommend Dr. Arnold Berman. He's excellent, as are his partners. Go there."

Why would I need a Neonatal Intensive Care Unit? I wondered, but I didn't ask. Looking back, I can't help but wonder if that was one of my first clues that, in fact, I didn't have a clue.

As a first-grade teacher, I gave and followed orders well. I was fortunate to get an appointment with Dr. Berman quickly, and while his office was further from home, the practice was a fabulous fit. I immediately felt a close connection with Dr. Berman and the nurses. At my 6-week appointment, I reported morning sickness. He confirmed that my nausea was normal, and I followed his instructions to eat a few saltines in bed before getting in the shower, sip carbonated drinks, and suck on ginger lozenges while at school. Despite the prophylactics, by my eighth week, I was very sick: vomiting every day along with chills and a low-grade fever at times. Dr. Berman was concerned. I had lost six pounds, which was substantial considering my already very small stature. After another week of watching the situation and my continued challenge holding down the food Jeff so lovingly prepared and forced upon me, I was admitted to the hospital. I stayed for four days on IV fluids to treat Hyperemesis Gravidarum, a big, scary term for severe nausea, vomiting, weight loss, and dehydration during pregnancy. I had never heard of it.

Beyond feeling physically awful, I was emotionally disturbed. I've never figured out what I did wrong to bring on the complication. Pregnancy was supposed to be vibrant and joyous, yet I was literally green and devoid of any joy whatsoever. I was terrified that the seed inside me stood no chance given the cyclone in my stomach. My job was to provide nutrition for my baby, and I wasn't getting it done. I wanted to grow the healthiest baby the doctors had ever seen. Dr. Berman met my paranoia and worry with massive reassurance that not only would I soon feel better but that I would also regain my weight plus more than I could imagine. He looked me in the eye and promised that by my 13th week, I would be a new woman. Like clockwork, my course corrected just as he guaranteed. Before I knew it, I was eating voraciously and not always sensibly. We've all heard of some interesting pregnancy cravings. Shamelessly, mine was Portillo's. Yep, a grilled hot dog with mustard, pickles, French fries, and a large Diet Coke. I limited the feast to three days a week, but boy, did I look forward to the 4 pm drive-thru after teaching. I was on my way! I put my early difficulties behind me and embraced the glory of my 2nd trimester, the honeymoon trimester as it's referred to. I delighted in the emergence of my (more than) bump and the flattering pregnancy courtesies I received. I would have been happy to spend the rest of my life just like that. It was, after all, a joyously expectant state. Right on cue, I started to feel fetal movement that wasn't gas. Check, check, check.

I relished my prenatal visits with Dr. Berman. There was no high greater than hearing my baby's heartbeat, like a watch ticking beneath a pillow. Or maybe there were: my ultrasound appointments. I couldn't get enough of his assurances that the heart rate and measurements were within normal range, perfect, actually. Not intending to burst my blissful bubble, Dr. Berman explained that there were two other doctors in the practice, and like many OB offices, I would meet with each of them over the last six weeks of my pregnancy. I didn't want to schedule appointments with the others because I liked Dr. Berman so much, trusted him, and needed *him* to deliver my baby. He explained the practice's policy in case he wasn't on call when I went into labor. I told him I'd like to know his call schedule, and that I'd find a way to make it work. He laughed; I was serious. I fought it as long as I could but eventually did meet the other two doctors and liked them well enough. Still, I wouldn't have it. Dr. Berman, my bestie, would deliver me, period.

Busy making lists, buying the supplies on the lists, and getting sad about leaving my students, I flew through my third trimester. Every aspect of my life was baby-ready. My classroom was ready to be handed over to a sub at any moment: the children's color-coded folders matched their respective lesson plans. Every label on every drawer was coordinated, and my notes to parents and colleagues covered more than they likely cared about. At home, the spice rack was alphabetized for my stand-in chef, outlets and cabinets were child-proofed, and the bills were paid with forward-dated checks and ready to be mailed.

Unable to process where the weeks had gone, I found myself at my 36-week appointment.

"Good news," Dr. Berman said.

"What?" I asked. "The baby's going to come out soon, and it's not going to hurt?"

"Sure," he laughed. "I know you'll be thrilled that we have a new doctor in the practice. He's going to pop in to . . ."

Before he could finish the sentence, there was a rap on the door. Dr. Berman looked to me to provide permission to enter.

In walked one of the most beautiful humans I have ever laid eyes on. I had a deep fondness for Italian food, leather, and pottery, but I hadn't before realized that I adore Italian men as well. His olive skin, shaggy black hair just over the ears, and white teeth (but not too white) on the tall, shapely body did me in. I sat there in my paper gown at the end of the exam table and suddenly felt faint. He was a physical specimen, perfect in every single way that I wasn't supposed to notice at eight months pregnant and happily married.

I was in love with him. It was that simple.

"Monica, this is Dr. Capezio," Dr. Berman said, breaking my trance.

"Oh, no, no, no," I exclaimed. "I know who you are, and you can't deliver my baby."

Dr. Capezio was spoken of among ladies of my age, mostly relative to his good looks. No one was talking about his academic research or surgical outcomes. He had attended Niles East High School, so he was local. His credentials were solid, yet I couldn't quite take him seriously. He was too hot. There was no way this man was going to see me writhing in the throes of labor and delivery, compromised.

"Thanks for stopping by," I said. "It was nice meeting you, but Dr. Berman will deliver my baby. You're way too cute, and I won't allow you to touch me."

"Oh-kay, Monica," he responded with a giggle. "We'll just chat then."

The three of us proceeded to talk for a few minutes, and I did warm up to him. He seemed like a compassionate medical professional. Even so, it was a non-starter. I explained to Dr. Berman that if there were a chance Dr. Capezio would deliver me that I'd have to leave the practice.

The very next week, I started to experience Braxton Hicks contractions. I called the practice every time to determine who was on call, even if it meant speaking to the answering service. It was my absolute obsession. Surely, I could fend off true labor until Dr. Berman was available. Control was my thing, and so I didn't get upset when the other docs were on; I just kept myself busy and stayed pregnant. Until I couldn't. My water broke in bed around 11 pm, so I had Jeff call the office to see who was on duty. We could drive to another hospital if need be. By the grace of God, Dr. Topel was on call, and I could live with that. He said to get there as soon as it was convenient but to take our time and get there safely.

We arrived at Lutheran General by midnight, and Dr. Topel remembered our conversation from the office visit and my desire for a natural birth, no drugs. He was committed to supporting me in that goal but did slip in that by far, the majority of women opted for epidurals. I was four centimeters dilated at the initial exam, pretty good progress for a first timer. As my discomfort swelled to agonizing pain, I was desperate for relief of any kind. I hadn't put any stake in funny breathing making a difference and therefore didn't pay too much attention in Lamaze class. Jeff, however, was a star student. He was steadfast in his desire to keep me out of pain and convinced me to follow along with him and the fancy breathing. The yoga ball and pressure point tricks didn't work either, and my mind wandered to drugs. No! I would prevail and be strong.

Around 4 am, Dr. Topol popped in to say goodbye.

"Wait, what?" I yelled. "What do you mean, you're leaving?!?!"

"Monica, it's the end of my shift," he explained. "While I wish I could deliver you, you know this is the way the practice works."

"Fine. When will Dr. Berman be here then?" I asked. He shook his head.

In walked my Italian Stallion. The shock was too much. The monitors caught my heart rate's acceleration, as he smiled big and tried not to laugh. He, too, was married. I think he just got a kick out of me.

"No, this isn't happening," I yelled again. I turned to Jeff and said, "Call the manager."

Dr. Capezio laughed and very calmly responded with "I'm going to deliver your child, Monica. I've got you. It's going to be a wonderful experience."

And it was, as soon as I begged him for every drug he could give me. I wanted epidural upon epidural and anything else he had up his sleeve or in the cabinet. From the moment Dr. Capezio assured me with his words and perfectly manicured hands and ordered my epidural, we were in perfect sync. He was my hero, and I would find a way to handle my passion for the man who was chief in command of my most private of parts (also perfectly manicured).

Thanks to Dr. Capezio, Stephanie Lynn joined us at 7:58 am on August 14, the new best day of my life. Sorry, Jeff. The love, hope, and promise I felt when she was handed to me surpassed the ecstasy of finding out I was pregnant. I would do anything and everything for this tiny human. Except, what was I supposed to do exactly?

Literally, everything was in order and ready, except for me.

In the hours and days that followed, my cluelessness glared. Never in a million years would I have shown up to class without a lesson plan; I was reputed to be the most prepared teacher at the school. But somehow, I showed up to motherhood without any sort of roadmap. The one thing I did know was that I was going to breastfeed. Nursing Stephie was not negotiable. It was how a mother passed along the perfect nutrients to her baby. Everyone knew that, even me. The pamphlets in the hospital goodie bag described that breastfed babies don't get cancer and are immune to all diseases. The nurses insinuated that breastfeeding meant a well-behaved child with a high IQ. And let's not forget the benefits to the mother, including decreased risk of breast and ovarian cancers. Conclusion: a mother owed it to her child (and herself) to breastfeed.

When it was time for discharge, I negotiated with the nurses to extend my stay. Stephie wasn't latching, and they knew all the positions to try. I needed their help and couldn't fathom going home. How was I going to feed her? Who would tell me what to do next?

Alas, I was kicked out of the hospital and reluctantly returned home. Nestled in my arms was the most beautiful cherub, yet magnificence was not what I saw, and peace was not what I felt. I sat slumped in the rocking chair: sweaty, swollen boobs hanging low to my still-bulging belly. I hardly recognized myself. Skin-to-skin contact, the nurses promised, would stimulate Stephie to nurse. It sounded far more romantic than it was. All I needed was the damn latch. It was all I could think about, my new obsession. I envisioned it every time I closed my eyes. I tried to recreate the illustrations in the brochures to no avail.

Why was Stephie not surrendering to primitive instinct? How did something so natural require nothing short of every star and meteor to align? I was desperate and abashedly shared my struggles with a dear friend. She offered some advice and a definitive solution.

"You're overthinking this, honey," Delphine said. "Here's what you'll do. Go into your bedroom alone with Stephie and close the door. Play some music. It's a beautiful day, and the sun is shining. Open the window just a crack and inhale the fresh air. Get undressed, relax on the bed, and position her at your nipple. Be sure to relax; that's important. You'll have an orgasm, maybe even more than one."

Umm, not quite. Here's what actually happened. After failing to relax (no big surprise) on the bed, I moved to the armchair in the corner for the back and elbow support. I took a deep breath, sat up straight, and optimistically aimed my left nipple at precisely the midpoint of Stephie's bottom lip like the nurse had shown me. Except, crap, it was supposed to be her top lip. I made the adjustment quickly, and her mouth began to open. Just as my nipple was positioned properly, her mouth clamped . . . empty. I held the tears, but my face flamed. I could do this! I had a freaking step-by-step guide. I moved through the listed actions as I would with my first graders or any good pie recipe.

Finally, after incessantly tickling her lips with my nipple, her mouth opened.

"Okay, Sweet Pea, this is it," I exclaimed.

I stuffed my nipple and entire areola right in there. She gazed past me, her eyes wide with surprise and bewilderment. I left it all in there for a few seconds, and there was nothing. No sucking, no swallowing.

"Sorry, Baby," I muttered and removed the mound of flesh from her petite mouth.

It hit me that I could have suffocated her with my gargantuan breast. She didn't seem to want it, and neither did I at that point. Stephie's endearing, soft fusses quickly mounted to ear-piercing shrieks for some g-d milk. I didn't blame her. My heart raced, my hands shook, and the tears came, along with the intrinsic panic of not being able to feed my baby. So much for the advice—we were on our own.

At that moment, I realized I might need to send her back. The decision to discharge her to my care looked like a lapse in competence or at least judgment. I had no business being a mother. Crushed, I returned to the nursery and laid her in the crib. I fell into the rocking chair, covered my ears, and ugly cried. I felt psychotic as I rocked back and forth, head between my knees, trying to ignore my and Stephie's bawling. Where was the promised deep bonding?

The chaos went on for days, even after my milk came in, and all the while, I wondered how Stephie was possibly getting the nutrition she needed. Jeff tried his best to appease my growing mania and bought a couple of breastfeeding books since I didn't have any. Everyone, including the pediatrician's office I had on speed dial, promised that babies eat what they need, but that wasn't our story. My breasts filled more and more, but she wasn't emptying them. Her patience had left the building, and I turned to the evil pump to both relieve my heavy breasts and to get something in her stomach. The torture device and pistons felt like penance for a job poorly done. The pain of my swollen breasts became unbearable, but Stephie would get the good stuff if it killed me.

Fifteen minutes of agony harvested intermittent yellowish-white drops totaling only a scant ounce from each hot and hard breast. It was difficult to feel proud, but I did at least feel responsible as I poured the liquid gold into a storage bag. My chapped nipples were stretched longer than I knew was possible. My breasts were wet and distorted to the shape of the pump's shield. I couldn't let Jeff see me. I looked and felt something short of human, like something of a bovine apparition.

Jeff was in a challenging spot, caught between supporting my crazed desire for Stephie to have breastmilk and advocating for my physical wellbeing. He was loyal to me and several times sheepishly suggested formula. I quickly vetoed the idea, and by the time my mother visited, I had a fever and couldn't lift either of my breasts to offer to Stephie. It was the worst pain I'd ever been in, and that's saying a lot so soon after having given birth with a fading epidural. Horrified by my state, my mother took matters into her own hands and called Dr. Berman. He asked a lot of questions, including whether I had tried pumping. It seemed I had done everything right.

His directive was clear and quick: "We need to stop the milk. Are you ready to stop?"

"Absolutely not, I can't stop breastfeeding," I said. "I need to nurse Stephie. What else can we do?"

"Monica, there's no gold medal, no trophy, for breastfeeding," he said. "You have mastitis, and I'm concerned about your fever and a bacterial infection. I'm also worried about how much Stephie *isn't* eating. What's important is keeping you healthy so that you can take care of your baby and keep her healthy."

Dr. Berman brought me down from my high expectations of myself and reset my perspective. "I know you were set on breastfeeding and that there is so much out there about 'breastfed is best,'" he said. "But I'm going on record to say, 'Fed is best.'" Not so patiently, yet professionally, he helped me see the options. My foremost responsibility was to keep Stephie alive, and to do that, I needed to feed her. I couldn't stay where and how I was for one minute longer. It was time to choose the right path forward. Jeff helped me see that this was a decision to be made based only on my and Stephie's needs and my doctor's advice . . . no one else's.

Reluctantly, but again desperate for pain relief, I agreed to follow Dr. Berman's recommendation. He called a prescription into the pharmacy and suggested Similac and Enfamil as two brands of formula that were nutritious and gentle on babies' stomachs. In what felt like a life-saving voyage, Jeff sped to Walgreens for baby formula and the medication to stop my milk production, STAT. It felt less appropriate than sending him out for tampons, but in the deepest parts of me, it also felt necessary.

Dr. Berman instructed my mother to bind me with cloth diapers. I will never forget the ceremony to flatten my breasts. She mummified me, wrapping me as tightly as she could. Relief came quickly, an effect of the compression even before the medication kicked in. Whenever the binding loosened, I begged her to tighten it. I went from a full C cup to an A cup, and the girls never bounced back. My breast tissue seemed to have been absorbed by my body along with the milk. Thank goodness for push-up bras.

Jeff and my mother fed Stephie her first couple of bottles of formula because it felt viscerally wrong to me. How could I give my baby fake milk? I watched from afar and slowly came closer to the scene. As I started feeling better physically, my mind cleared as well. I realized that I had actually saved Stephie. I saved her from myself and my rigid notion of how I should feed her. I saved her from my cluelessness that legitimate, even good, alternatives existed. There is almost always another option in life, and it's up to us to stay open to those options.

From the time Stephie started eating as voraciously as I had eaten my Portillo's, we made drastic improvements, and I came to look forward to feeding her. The reward of her satisfaction was intense, and the ensuing milk coma was the cherry on top. Recording how many ounces she ate at each feeding felt so good to my organized mind. It was tremendously reassuring to know that she was getting enough. I dare say I was becoming slightly capable. I slowly allowed myself to love her, to be infatuated with her.

With the feeding issues resolved, I expected to reclaim my life, but sleep deprivation, a general sadness, and the stress of Stephie's new projectile vomiting and colic brought ongoing pandemonium instead. If she was awake, she was crying. As soon as I cleaned her up and changed my own rancid clothes, we did it all again. Our pediatrician wasn't concerned because Stephie was gaining weight. She assured me that her digestive system was just immature and that the eruptions would end in time. While I waited, I was to use gas drops, burp her every ounce or two, and prop her up for 15 minutes after feeding. It wasn't supposed to be so complicated, so unnatural. Why were babies born before they were mature enough to eat properly anyway?

The nights were disproportionately long, like recurring scenes from *Where the Wild Things Are*. I wanted Jeff to sleep so he'd be clear for work in the mornings. But he was often awakened by the shrieks—always Stephie's and sometimes mine. One night in particular is emblazoned in my mind. I never went to bed. Between warming and feeding bottles, pacing the house (but, in fact, not quieting Stephie), and cleaning up after explosions from both ends, there was no time for sleep. By 2 am my pajama drawer was empty, its contents scattered across the house, and I'd tapped into my nicer nighties. Jeff kept checking on us, but I held him off, wanting to do my job myself.

Clueless with a Capital "C"

"Monnie, let me help you. You need a break," he encouraged. "Go change and take a shower. You look good, though!"

Confused, I touched my crusty hair and scanned the rest of me. I stood, zombie-like, in a lacey little number I hadn't worn since our honeymoon. Jeff chuckled, but I couldn't.

Nights were the worst, but the days were also confusing, scary, and untethered. For an individual who thrives on control and predictability, it was hell. I couldn't help wondering if Stephie would be vomiting and crying so violently if she were consuming my milk, the milk nature intended for her. My dear mother would come to the house each morning at 6 o'clock to hold or feed Stephie so I could sleep or clean myself. Only when my mother was with Stephie could I really rest because I knew we were both safe. It was the only time I didn't hear phantom cries in my head. My mother was my savior. While I appreciated the help, it drew attention to my inability to do motherhood without my own mother. What was wrong with me?

Even with the privileged service of my loving mother and husband, I didn't leave the house for the first three months of Stephie's life. I was too emotional and physically exhausted. Too much could go wrong. In short, I wasn't fit for the public, especially a public that expected to see the same Monica I had always been. That woman was lost temporarily and not available to me or others.

Something shifted around the three-month mark. Stephie's little baby body did mature, as predicted. She started to sleep for good chunks at night and was predictably sleeping for three naps during the day. As her GI system matured, my nervous system calmed. Naptime was always a debate between sleeping myself or doing something that I couldn't do when she was awake. I challenged myself to choose the latter. I would prepare dinner or bake my favorite chocolate chip cookies, which conjured a glimmer of the Monica I used to know—a functional, capable human being who did more than react to biological messes. The photos in Stephie's baby book begin at three months.

It would be many years before I could let go of my shame and see my cluelessness for what it was: normal, expected First-timer's Syndrome. It's hard to perform perfectly the first time one does anything, regardless of best intentions, responsible preparations, and heartfelt efforts. My hospitalization early in pregnancy, failure to execute a natural delivery, inability to nurse, limited skill in quieting Stephie, and my deep dependency on Jeff and my mother were scorched in my mind. I hadn't recalled that I hadn't always been competent in the other areas of my life. For instance, it took me a full semester to adjust to the rigors of college. My pupils gave me a run for it during my first few weeks of student teaching, and Jeff told me it took a couple months before I became a good roommate. But I had forgotten all of that.

Memories of my early motherhood still bring embarrassment, but I've learned to have compassion for the person I was. It wasn't until I was asked to recount this story that I recognized just how hard I was on myself and the resultant pain. I truly believed I was clueless and incompetent and didn't toss myself any grace for what I was experiencing and up against as a new mother, a first timer. Believe it or not, I'm just now deciphering that what I saw as clueless and incompetent was actually to be expected. That's what I was *actually* clueless about! It's normal for a new mother to feel that way, as if her life has been pulled out from under her, leaving an existence that is foreign and hard to navigate.

39 years ago feels like last week, and I'll be a grandmother soon. Stephie, my high-achieving formula-fed baby, is expecting! I'm committed to helping her have compassion for herself as a new mother by sharing my experience. She'll get to determine whether it's wisdom, but at the very least, she will hear my truth. I want Stephie to be educated and prepared in a way I was not.

I may have held one baby prior to Stephie. I didn't have family, friends, or teaching peers who had babies, and my own mother didn't talk to me about mothering. I want Stephie to expect that there will be hardships, anticipate that they will pass, and know that a new normal will set in. I will tell her not to compare her new life to the one she used to lead because they aren't comparable. I will encourage Stephie as gently as possible to go easy on and take care of herself so she can in turn take the best care possible of her baby. I've heard it said that grandmotherhood is even better than motherhood. I can hardly believe the claim, and I definitely can't wait for the next chapter.

Chapter 4

Bikinis, Barbies, and Christmas Pizza

AIMEE

"Don't compare yourself. There is no comparison between the sun and the moon. They shine when it's their time."

—Anonymous

A glance in the mirror can be quick or prolonged, literal or figurative, trite or profound, complimentary or critical, depending on the day. We don't often commit these glances to memory or hold onto them as a compass. A photograph, however, is documentation of history, ongoing evidence of how things once were. The history itself doesn't change, of course, but our perspective on it can. That's the power of a picture.

When I think back to my first months of motherhood, my mind jumps to a photo with Grant, my firstborn of four boys. We were at one of my favorite places on the planet, Door County, Wisconsin, a true sanctuary for my soul with its beaches, winding roads, lighthouses, and sunsets. My mother was the photographer. From behind the camera, she exclaimed, "You look so beautiful and sexy." I was confused. Was she talking to me? I certainly didn't feel sexy as I stood at the edge of Lake Michigan, Grant on my hip. I wore a pink patterned one-piece swimsuit and stood at an angle to mask my postpartum curves. Okay, curves sound attractive. But to me, at that point in my life, they were anything but. I wanted to cover myself and reduce my exposure. I figured I'd never wear a bikini again.

With the clarity of hindsight, I *do* see it. Perhaps not *Sports Illustrated Swimsuit* material, but not so bad after all. The sunshine aside, I was radiant. My body had grown Grant, birthed him, and fed him for five months, for a total of 14 months of service to the lad. What a miraculous feat. Now when I hold the photo, my eyes zip right past the swimsuit and land hard on my facial expression. There isn't a singular adjective to describe it. It was one of intimacy and fierce love. My professional wedding photos don't come close to such a candid, deep, and genuine look in my eyes and glow from within. Beyond love, the moment bundled pride, splendor, and a tad bit of naivete. I wish I could've seen what my mom saw that day, but I couldn't. I compared myself to my pre-pregnancy, pre-motherhood body and self. I see how that was unfair now, but I didn't have my head on quite right then. Thanks to physical and emotional exhaustion, I felt like I was constantly treading water, gasping for oxygen right at the surface. I couldn't stop kicking and flailing, or I would surely drown. That's likely why I remember that trip so fondly. Eric, Grant, and I were on vacation with my parents, and I was surrounded by willing and helpful hands, if only for a few days. I temporarily came up for air and truly enjoyed my days with my newly expanded family.

From the time I was a young girl, I envisioned myself as a mother. I wanted lots of babies, as in five or six. Going into motherhood, I knew I'd be tired and that sleep would be fleeting.

That expectation was properly set. But no person or book prepared me emotionally for those early days and months. My new role felt natural, like it was meant to be, but it also felt hard and strange. Human nature predisposes us to fit into a framework, definition, or paradigm. Becoming a mother ignited in me a whole new variety of self-evaluation and comparison. Each day delivered new challenges, and I so badly wanted to make sense of my experiences.

From my living room window where I nursed Grant, I watched my neighbor, Mae, head out on picnics and other adventures with her three kids when I could barely make it to Target with my one. *Why couldn't I do more? I used to get through my daily to-do list with no problem. Why was I less qualified than Mae to get everything done?* In those questions, I was caught in the traps of comparison and reminded constantly that I was falling behind.

I learned in the course of having four baby boys that there are good comparisons and bad comparisons. A good comparison can raise our awareness of what we want for ourselves, remind us of our highest potential, and guide us in getting there. In contrast, bad comparisons place an emphasis on external feedback and threaten what we intrinsically know is good or right for ourselves.

As I reflect on my early motherhood journey, I see segments of a film reel or episodes of a Netflix drama series. I hope you will find comfort, self-compassion, and maybe even a laugh or two in what follows.

PILOT: Domestic Queen

Let's start with a good comparison, and I'll use my own dear mother as an example. Although not palatial, our childhood home was lovely in every way. Mom always made us feel special, cooking healthy meals and wrapping us in bear hugs. She was my model, a perfect mother. Even more so now that she's gone, I hold her on an opulent and very high pedestal. Naturally, I committed myself to her same standards.

Mom was a domestic queen and dedicated herself fully to Dad, me, and my two brothers when we were young. Eventually, she returned to a tenured teaching career, continuing her deep need for service and stewardship. She did it all. When Eric and I got married, I channeled her. *What would Mom serve for dinner on a chilly Wednesday night in November? Would Mom iron this shirt or send it to the dry cleaner?* I wanted to be the perfect wife. And then at the age of 29, I wanted to be the perfect stay-at-home mother with perfect clothes, a perfect home, a perfect marriage, and a perfectly-cared-for-son. The need for everything and everyone (most notably myself) to be clean and to have dinner on the table for Eric when he was in town was intense. It didn't change because I had a newborn or because Eric traveled extensively on business. Nope, Grant was a new and incremental responsibility, not a swapped one. I learned to save my shower for as late in the day as possible because who knew what the day had in store? Bouts of stomach upset? Crawling in the dirt at the park? Playing in the sand? It just made sense to wait as there wasn't always time for two showers with a little one.

I would pick up the house when Grant slept. I didn't abide by the rule of sleeping when the baby sleeps. I understand the theory and don't judge anyone who does follow it, but it wasn't an option for me. If I had slept when Grant had slept, I wouldn't have gotten anything done, and that just wasn't okay with me. There were always calls to return, bills to pay, and laundry to wash, fold, or put away. It was really, really hard when he was little. Naps were unpredictable and typically much shorter than I appreciated. Many times, I didn't complete a single task, and I would sometimes resent the initial grunts of his waking and the interruption of my productivity. It often seemed impossible that he could need to eat again so soon. The race against the clock was perpetual.

There were days following sleepless nights when it was tempting to nap with Grant. I can count on one hand how many times it happened, though, because I had a choice: to sleep or to keep up. I couldn't do both, so I consistently chose to keep up. After putting him down in the evening, I collected the sticky, crusty burp clothes, blankets, and clothing, ran the vacuum, emptied and restocked the diaper bag, and cleaned the kitchen. Early on, he might wake up for a final feeding just as I was finishing my housework. There were no breaks. As he got a little older, Grant slept into the night. All along the way, however, I couldn't go to sleep myself with the house a mess. It's just the way I'm wired. I chose to keep up because when it was finally time to turn off the light, I could do so with a clear conscience. My standards didn't bend just because I had a baby. My mom did it all, and that's how I would do it, too. I didn't process the self-imposed pressure at the time.

S1 EPISODE 1:
Over-the-Shoulder-Boulder-Holder

I thrived on reporting in with the pediatrician and gaining his approval of Grant's weight gain and development. I logged every feeding and diaper change. Even now, I love laughing at the notes I made. Even if my handwriting was illegible by night, my conviction to record all that happened (and get a gold star for it) was strong. No matter what the previous day and night held, early mornings were a blessed and hopeful part of my days.

Morning runs have always been an outlet for me, and I held tight to them through all my babies. Whether or not I had gone back to sleep following overnight feedings, I would head out on a run or for a swim by 5:30 am before Eric left for work. It was my chance to be in my own head, move my body in a forward motion at a quick clip, and snatch the endorphins that would sustain me through the day. I didn't exercise to get my body back. I ran or swam because it gave me more energy and more vitality in caring for the boys. I didn't always want to go, but I was very disciplined and always felt better as soon as I got moving. It was one of the few things I did for myself back then, 30 to 60 minutes that fed my survival. If I was better, I could serve the boys better.

Grant was seven months old when my mom called one morning on her way to school. "Honey, you really need a more supportive sports bra," she said. "I saw you running down Green Bay Road." I made a mental note to change my route.

Mom didn't beat around the bush. She told it the way it was, which I appreciated most of the time. I knew she was trying to help, but my sleep-deprived feelings were hurt. It took all of me to just get out there and hit some semblance of a stride in the very tight time window I had between feedings. My breasts often felt like boulders as I ran, but I didn't think much of it. Until Mom's well-intended feedback translated to this: *Aimee's a mess. Her boobs are at her chin one second and her belly button the next. One's a lot bigger than the other, and the left one is leaking.*

The message would have rolled off during any other period of my life. But again, sleep deprivation. If my own mother saw me as a hot mess, I wondered how others saw me. That contemplation didn't cross my mind the first few weeks postpartum because my brain worked only for Grant, for my body's production of sustenance for him, and my strong will to keep my eyes open. I didn't have the capacity to care what anyone but Grant thought of me. But as I started to leave the house for quick trips to the grocery store, I started looking around and noticing other mothers and babies. They didn't have dark circles under their eyes. I wondered if they were as tired as I was, and I wondered what type of bras they wore. My meandering mind sought context for my own experience. How did other active moms juggle nursing and exercise? It was stuck in a cycle of comparison, this time to other mothers, and it took me to deep, dark places. One day it took me to the mall. Cue the bad kind of comparison.

S1 EPISODE 2: Barbies

It was too hot outside to take Grant for a stroll, and I desperately needed new underwear (including a sports bra, apparently) and mascara. So, I took the opportunity to head to the mall. I'd be in and out of Macy's before Grant had time to notice. I pulled into the "Expectant/New Mother" parking space but didn't feel very VIP-y. It was the first time I'd used the Snap-n-Go stroller, and I struggled with the red "release" buttons. The entire point of the contraption was that it was a breeze to use. I felt the jeers of fellow shoppers making their way to the entrance. *Other moms could unfold and operate their strollers. Why couldn't I figure it out? In that moment, doing something for myself and taking care of Grant simultaneously started to feel like a conflict of interest. I should have just stayed home.* Flustered, I called on my angels for help. Within a couple minutes, I had Grant's car carrier securely snapped in place and the diaper bag stowed in the basket below. I tousled my hair, adjusted my posture, and headed in. The A/C raged, and poor Grant sprouted goosebumps immediately. Dressed for the weather, Grant was in a onesie, and I was wearing a nursing tank and a pair of shorts that were newly tight. I should have remembered that malls, movie theaters and churches always overdo the air conditioning. I instinctively untied the cardigan around my waist (meant to hide the tight shorts) and tucked it around Grant. We were only minutes in, and the outing didn't seem worth it. I wanted to abort the mission, fade away back to the car, and disappear from the scene altogether.

Never before had I noticed the flocks of women and strollers congregated at storefronts and eateries. Had the population always been there, and I hadn't noticed? Or had I not actually been to a mall on a weekday morning because I'd been at work? In any case, I was taken aback. The fenced off treehouse play area was packed with perfectly coiffed, Barbie-like, young mothers, all with Starbucks cups in-hand . . . and a couple of nannies. The mothers were engaged in smiley conversation with the mothers, and the nannies with the nannies . . . the kind of cliques we all remember from junior high. I overheard the mom closest to me talking about how her 8-week-old was sleeping through the night. I called BS in my head, but the other gal nodded and said hers was sleeping well, too. Their babies weren't crying and if they smelled like poop or vomit, I couldn't smell it from across the fence. *Why wasn't Grant sleeping through the night? What were they doing that I wasn't?* I didn't have time to figure it out. I needed caffeine.

I hit Macy's makeup counter and lingerie department with a double espresso in hand and couldn't resist swinging through the children's department. Grant needed absolutely nothing. We had clothes in every size and for every season, and I was still writing thank-you notes for all the baby gifts. Still, it was fun to scan the sale rack. There was a group of three moms with strollers a couple racks over. They were seriously everywhere! They must have been besties from high school who'd planned their pregnancies together. They didn't notice me as I unintentionally eavesdropped.

"Who's in love with their stroller?" one of them asked. "I don't like the one I registered for. Stu will kill me, but I really want to get a different one."

"I love my Peg Perego for the mall or the zoo," another responded. "I have a jogger, too, for longer, faster walks around the neighborhood. It's too hard to put in the car, though, and it takes up so much space in the garage. I have an umbrella stroller for when he's a little bigger, but I don't know what I'll use that one for. Strollers are kind of my new handbags."

"I wonder if it comes in a double stroller," the first one said. "If I'm going to spend that much, it would be nice if Mason could ride too when he's tired or at least stand on one of those platform thingies on the back."

"Speaking of Mason," the third one chimed in. "Which preschool is he at? I need to get Clementine on a few waiting lists."

"He's in the Presby toddler class," she said. "They take them at 18-months. Definitely apply there for the morning program."

I felt nauseous. Since my friends didn't have children yet and I hadn't made new friends in the neighborhood, posh strollers and preschool decisions weren't at the top of my mind. I definitely didn't relate. I was on the practical side when it came to strollers, diaper bags, and clothing. High-end brands weren't my thing, and there was no way I'd be sending Grant to school when he was still a baby! I was the odd one out.

A few moans from Grant snapped me out of the chatter in my head. He was hungry—time to get moving. I hightailed it out of Macy's but got distracted by the music coming from Gymboree, one of those hands-on play studios for parents, babies, and toddlers. I paused at the entrance. Several of the books I was reading emphasized the need to socialize your baby early, especially if he wasn't going to be in a daycare environment. I understood the benefit to Grant, but I couldn't do it. I'd repeatedly made excuses for why I couldn't make it to the playgroup my neighbor kept inviting me to. I imagined circles of comparison and expected that I'd be judged for what Grant was wearing and eating and how he was behaving. Maybe even what toys we had. I didn't care how others were doing things, and I wasn't looking for unsolicited commentary about how I was doing them.

Comparison was everywhere when I went out into the world, and at times it crept into the territory of judgment. I see now that comparison hurt me in more ways than one. It caused me to put so much pressure on myself, and it also kept me separate from those I was comparing myself to. It drove a wedge. I assumed that was what mommy groups were about. But I never went, so I guess I didn't actually know. Maybe they were the sweetest women I never knew. Society sets enough impossible expectations on us, and if we could just ditch the trap of comparison, we could lean on each other better. After all, we're all Barbies, regardless of things like hair color, waist size, and occupation. Maybe the Barbies on the other side of the fence that day were helping each other see themselves as the powerful people we mothers all are.

S1 EPISODE 3: Left to My Own Devices

If Eric and I had the chance to go out to dinner when he was in town, I knew Mom's response would be "Find a babysitter." Right out of the gate, she made clear that she would babysit on exactly two occasions: if she wanted to and in an emergency. Her staunch stipulations surprised and hurt me, and it was clear she wouldn't budge from them. But when Oakley, our black lab, had a seizure one evening when Eric was gone, I expected the circumstance would fit her "emergency" proviso. Oakley had defecated, urinated, and vomited all over the kitchen, and I couldn't sanitize the kitchen *and* tend to Grant. He didn't like to be put down when he was awake. I probably created my own monster as I'd become adept at loading the washing machine and dryer with one hand while I nursed him in the other arm.

Oakley was my first baby and so more than the mess, I wanted to take care of him, to comfort him and to hold him. I needed help, and my heart was torn between my babies, so naturally, I called my mother.

"Mom, I need you. I need to take Oakley to the emergency vet," I said, explaining the mess. "I'll feed Grant now, and can you come to bathe him and get him to bed while I deal with this?"

"So sorry to hear about Oakley," she said. "I'll send your dad over to help with the dog. Good luck."

I rallied and got through the immediate disaster on my own, but I was in shock and felt totally abandoned and confused. I mean, my mom and I were close. We spoke multiple times a day, and she was wonderful with Grant when she came to visit. But the stake was in the ground back then . . . no babysitting. My aunt helped my cousin when her kids were young, and I figured my mom would do the same for me. I believe my continued hardship in asking *anyone* for help is a consequence of my being burned by asking my mother for help. After all, if I asked my own mother and she said no, why would anyone else say yes?

I gave my mom the benefit of the doubt most times. She was still working full-time and was probably trying to establish reasonable boundaries. Maybe it was her way of saying to me, "You have a child now. You're going to raise your own child; I'm not going to do it for you." Over the years, she was warm with all my boys and developed special relationships with each one. Honestly, I still try to make sense of it. The stance was so contrary to her other copious points of support for me . . . and so detached. Maybe it will crystallize when I become a grandmother myself one day, but I kind of doubt it. I expect I'll want to be very involved and help however I can, assuming my daughters-in-law will have me.

S1 EPISODE 4: Diana's Resort

To the rescue came one Friday's phone call from a former work friend, Diana. She had received Grant's birth announcement and wanted to reconnect. I'd always valued Diana as that co-worker we all count on to make long afternoons in Cube City, and lunch breaks, a little more enjoyable. We were close, despite the gap in our ages. I think our friendship worked so easily for two reasons.

First, I had always been on the mature side for my age. Second, I think Diana saw a lot of herself in me.

We picked up right where we had left off, and the conversation quickly leapt to my new world. She asked all the right questions, and I provided all the right answers.

"How in the world did you push out 9 pounds 4 ounces worth of baby?" she asked.

"That's a story for a glass of wine or two," I laughed.

She inquired about Grant's temperament and our day-to-day activities. "Yes, Grant's a wonderful baby, easy," I said. "Yes, I'm 100% positive about my decision to stay home with him. It's all I've ever wanted."

Everything was in the affirmative. We were fine. Everything was fine. No discombobulation here! We talked for nearly an hour while Grant napped, and we got all caught up on her sons, her husband, and her pursuit of a personal training certification.

Diana must have sensed something in my responses, something beyond my words. She knew me well and must have picked up on my flat tone or general lack of spark. I wasn't overtly floundering. In fact, I didn't think I was floundering at all, even privately. By that point, I'd figured out mothering was hard, but I wasn't going to admit to anyone just how hard it was. Before we hung up, she asked if I'd like to bring Grant to her house on Monday. I was surprised. She said she'd fill up the kiddie pool she still had in the garage and that she'd make lunch for us, and we could eat out on the porch.

"Thanks so much, Diana, really," I said. "But Grant will need to nap, and he's a cluster feeder. Maybe I could take a raincheck for this fall or winter?"

"Aimee, Honey, I'll take care of everything," she said. "I'll get Max's old crib out, and Grant can sleep in there. Feed him whenever you need to. Please, let me spoil you."

She twisted my arm, and I spent the entire afternoon at her welcoming home. The acreage and her hospitality were like a fine resort. Diana coddled me; she cared for me that day in ways no one else had in my time as a mother. Letting someone wait on me felt strange, but it also felt lovely. That Friday call and that Monday visit brought Diana and me back together as friends, personal friends this time. She dutifully checked in with me every few weeks and called me out when I dishonestly answered one of her questions. She encouraged me to tell her the truth. She had been through exactly what I was facing years before with her own children. She had lived it, survived it, and was willing to talk about it. She talked about what was hard for her and asked me what was hardest for me. I told her how I couldn't stop comparing myself to my former self, other mothers, and my own mother.

Each conversation with Diana was like a breath of fresh air. I'll never forget her words one day: "You have this idea of who other moms are and what they do. They aren't perfect, Aimee." Diana was my voice of reason, and her comment gave me promising perspective. I committed to her that I would try to compare myself less.

S1 EPISODE 5: The Sputtering Spigot

When better for the A/C to break than the dog days of summer in the Midwest? The local media was having a heyday that week, reporting record-setting temperatures and running segments on cooling shelters for vulnerable populations, including the elderly and the homeless. Grant and I might as well have shown up for a bed. The porch thermometer registered 102°F in the shade, and the air in the house was stagnant with the exception of strategically placed oscillating fans. I was sweating buckets, and Grant was crying and crying and crying, which got me crying and crying and crying. I repeatedly checked his diaper. Although hot and sweaty, he didn't have a fever. Could he be teething so early? I was at a complete loss as to why he was inconsolable.

I broke down and called Dr. Klein. He asked me tons of questions, and we agreed that Grant didn't seem ill. That was a relief. But then, what was the problem? Dr. Klein changed the line of questioning to focus on Grant's feeding schedule. I had specific answers, per my logs.

"Has he always cried at the end of a feeding?" he asked.

"No, almost never," I said. "He either falls asleep or is ready to play."

"Okay, I think I know what's going on," he said. "I think he's still hungry."

"What do you mean?" I asked. "He's eating like eight times a day, so I don't know how he could be hungry."

"Aimee, Grant's a big boy," he reminded me. "You're doing an amazing job feeding him, but I think your milk supply just isn't keeping up with his need for so much milk right now."

I was crushed. Grant was starving, and I couldn't produce what he needed. The spigot was sputtering, and I wouldn't let the well go dry. Dr. Klein's comment felt like a direct accusation of my inadequacy. It wasn't intended as such, but that's how I took it. He went on to tell me I could supplement with formula while continuing to nurse Grant. *Did other moms supplement? I thought you either breastfed or bottle fed.* I'd read that supplementing could interfere with my own milk supply, but we couldn't go on like we were. Dr. Klein was convincing in his encouragement to use formula, so I put my pride aside and gave Grant his first bottle later that day. It felt strange feeding him powdered milk, but he was so happy. That's all I wanted. Fortunately, his cries forced me to open my mind to alternatives, and supplementing was a godsend for both of us.

SEASON FINALE: Christmas Pizza

We'd recently moved to Madison, Wisconsin, where I knew no one and was truly removed from everything. I was on an island that wasn't tropical and sunny, and there was no cabana boy. I had all four boys at that point, and Gage (the youngest) was an infant. It was Christmastime, the most wonderful time of the year. Only it wasn't. Late afternoons/early evenings with any child, let alone four children under 6 years old, were rough. I'd fed the older boys and had just sat down to nurse Gage and watch the 5:30 pm news, trying to keep a pulse on what was happening outside of our cocoon. Notwithstanding the new house, my healthy, happy (most of the time) children, the fresh-cut tree in the living room, and the light snow falling outside, I completely broke down over an Infinity commercial. You know, the ones where the husband gifts the wife a car with a big red bow on top.

My unhappiness shone brighter than any bulb on the tree. It was Christmas, and I wasn't happy. Why, I wondered. It wasn't about a shiny new SUV, and I had everything else going for me. It didn't make sense that I felt so sad and alone in the company of my four boys. I got everyone to bed, cleaned up the dinner and playroom messes, and sat back down. Maybe the problem was sitting down, stopping, and actually processing a complete thought. I reviewed the long gift list I wanted to manifest for the boys. I had the grocery lists of turkey for Christmas Eve, tenderloin for Christmas Day, and everything that went along with the main courses. And then there was the fact that I hadn't been shopping for myself in at least a year and didn't have anything contemporary in my closet to wear to church or my mom's house. The mountain of to-do's was always high, but at Christmastime it got to the point of insurmountable, and it started to feel more like a volcano about to erupt than your run-of-the-mill mountain. Eric still traveled all the time, so I called Diana.

"Diana, I think I'm losing it. All I want to do is curl up in a ball and cry," I said. "This is supposed to be the best time of the year, especially with little kids. It's supposed to be precious."

"Oh, Sweetie. Says who?" she asked. "There are two issues here. First, motherhood is damn hard, and you've been doing it alone. You're keeping four small humans alive. You're doing it on three hours of sleep a night, and you're doing it alone. You're amazing."

"Thanks for saying that, but I think it's what every mother does," I said. "I'm nothing special in the mother department, and I feel totally in a fog."

"Wrong-o. Not every mother does it the way you do it, to the level you do it," she said. "The second thing is Christmas, Shmitmas. Christmas hoopla is a farce if you're comparing your own to what you see on TV. I know it's hard to ignore TV, catalogs, and movies. We have to be honest here. It's not all ribbons and bows. Sure, there are nice moments, but Christmas also comes with endless expectations, superficial celebrations, and no time for ourselves."

"I guess I don't know what Christmas is to me," I said. "I thought I knew that it was beautifully wrapped packages, jubilant children, and dining tables set with China and crystal. Fantasy, I guess."

"Aimee, you can't be everything," Diana said. "You can't be in an apron and high heels basting the turkey, keeping the kids safe, all while being a doting wife. The time and energy required simply don't exist. You might think you *want* that, but you don't *need* that. Do yourself a favor and forget about what you see and what Christmas was like as a kid. Make a list of what you want Christmas to be for *your* family."

I couldn't help but wonder why Eric or my mother wasn't making these suggestions to me. Eric had other things like building our bank account and advancing his career on his mind and therefore didn't consider how it would be to be in my shoes. With my mom, I think sometimes mothers and daughters are so close that mothers don't fully see what their daughters are going through. Diana was almost the mom to me that my mom couldn't be in some respects. But I didn't get hung up on that.

Instead, I wrote the list: #1 Real happiness, #2 Peace, and #3 Joy. I knew what *wouldn't* yield those things: frantic shopping for the next 10 days, gift wrapping by night, or comparison to how new neighbors, friends, and family members "did" Christmas. Diana gave me permission to "do our family" and to let go of comparison.

So, I focused on the kids and pushed aside the notion of gourmet meals. I took it so seriously that we ordered pizzas on Christmas Eve and gave the older kids root beer from the gas station. I was worried Eric would be disappointed, but I think the reduction of my own stress served him well. It was some of the best pizza I've ever had. We skipped church and prayed for forgiveness. We watched Rudolph and managed to accomplish all three things on my list. I won't lie and say it didn't feel a little rogue, but more than that, it felt free. Free from norms, free from "I should's," and free from false pretenses of who our family was. That year's replacement of dress clothes with cozy Christmas pajamas (before matching Christmas PJs were a thing) warms my heart each time I come across the photos.

ROLLING CREDITS

Future episodes and seasons of my motherhood were informed by the cast and events of Season 1. I'm grateful for all my experiences, especially the challenging ones that forced me to be brave and think in new capacities (about myself, my babies, and other mothers). As I became more experienced with subsequent babies, things got easier. Not easy, but easier. Even so, I had to remind myself to be cautious of comparison: comparison of my new self to my old self, comparison of how I mothered vs. how others mothered, and comparison of my life to what others' lives looked like from the outside. The inclination to compare is natural because it feels like a data point. Therein lies the danger: it's incomplete data and faulty feedback. We have to be careful about letting anyone or anything other than ourselves inform our sense of success and worthiness as mothers.

My comparison of myself to my mother stretched me and made me better than I may have otherwise strived to be. I reached higher heights thanks to her. That comparison was productive. Hard and humbling at times, but net positive. I'm proud of who I am as a mother, and that is a lot to do with my own mother's ways.

On the contrary, my comparison of myself to other mothers and of my babies to other babies was not productive. It resulted in unnecessary pain. It's easy to reach the conclusion that everyone else is one way, doing things one way, and that you're different. This can result in loneliness, isolation, and self-doubt. Maybe that seemingly perfect mother is pulling her hair out or downing a bottle of Chardonnay by night. There is always a behind-the-scenes, and that's true for life, marriage, family, work, etc. It's fruitless to compare apples to oranges or the sun to the moon.

With due respect for what I thought and felt at the time, today, I'm not intimidated when I choose to do things differently from others. I don't feel defensive, insecure, or scared of my choices. We can—and should—learn from each other as mothers. We need peers and people who have lived through it, who are a little savvier and a little calmer (people like Diana) to tell us to "do you." If we heard that message more, then we could enjoy the baby snuggles more.

Before I wrap, I need to issue one admittance. I attended (and enjoyed) a mom-and-tot class at an institution called Wiggle

Worms. Are you laughing? I believe my enjoyment stemmed from these factors in particular: 1) The class was structured and featured a teacher, therefore not allowing much time for catty conversation amongst the mothers; 2) Grant clearly enjoyed the interaction with other babies, and his coos and outreached arms brought me joy; 3) The class took place a couple towns away from ours, so Grant and I could show up incognito; and 4) The once a week meeting served the dual purpose of socializing Grant and getting me out of the house. It fit well between naps, which was always a requirement of my regimented days.

While I didn't make friends per se at Wiggle Worms, it was indeed a community centered on mutual respect of the trials and tribulations of motherhood. I see now how important that was. If you haven't heard Gloria's monologue from the 2023 *Barbie* movie, please get your hands on it. I will always be grateful for the sisterhood it inspires. Despite differences in our individual circumstances, we're all in the same good fight. We fight to be true to ourselves as women [and mothers] and support each other in knowing that we're not only good, but great, just the way we are.

As my boys grew, I was very involved with their activities and took on leadership roles at their schools. I worked with mothers of many flavors, opinions, and backgrounds. As I recognized my tendency to compare myself, I knew I needed to protect myself by *not* doing it. I'm not a loner, but I do choose my company carefully. I do things my way that works for me and my boys. And to this day, you'll find me watching little league baseball games from the comfort and solitude of the outfield. You should try it sometime! Just remember to bring your own refreshments because concessions aren't served out there.

I figured it wrong back then. In fact, today I wear only bikinis. One-piece swimming suits make me feel frumpy. I'm proud of my curves and the other artifacts of my pregnancies. I wear the bikini for myself and no one else. If it happens to inspire a glance, I guess I'll take it. What matters is how *I* feel when I look in the mirror on my way to paddleboard or to meditate at the beach. Because how I look today reflects all that I've become as a mother and all I've given in that role. And yes, I have time to paddleboard and meditate these days. You will, too!

Chapter 5

To Thine Own Self be True

SARA

"To all the girls who no longer believe in fairytales or happy endings: You are the writer of this story. Chin up and straighten your crown. You're the queen of this kingdom and only you know how to rule it.

—B. Devine

As girls, we're shown knights in shining armor gallantly rescuing damsels in distress. We see princesses marrying princes in ornately clad castles and riding into the sunset. As women, we're left to reconcile our lives' experiences to those of fairytales. The illusions and romanticism continue beyond marriage to how babies arrive to us and how they enhance us. My happily ever came *after* a seven-year fertility journey. *After* acupuncture, eight rounds of IVF, 300 injections, two stillbirths, and a miscarriage. *After* my mother delivered my baby. And *after* I learned to mother according to my own North Star and no one else's.

Oh, you caught that detail about my mother having my baby? Sounds like science fiction, right? Here's how it happened. My husband Bill and I were beaming, fulfilled in our young marriage, and working jobs that we loved. We were ready to be parents. Yet, my period showed up all too reliably for months after I'd stopped popping the pill, and despite our best maneuvers. How could this be? I treated my body as a holy land, ingesting only the cleanest, most nutritious foods. I'd switched to organic skincare and cleaning products. I hadn't taken Advil in 10 years. I should have been ripe for breeding.

At my acupuncturist's direction, I brewed syrupy herbal teas from scratch. Bill and I sprayed our room with essential oils, and I placed a fertility goddess statue next to our bed, a gift from a friend who'd had four children. Initial frustration intensified to panic when two years of holistic treatment yielded nothing, and my gynecologist recommended that I see a reproductive endocrinologist. There were tests, so many tests. An MRI revealed Empty Sella, a pituitary gland condition resulting in the insufficient firing of various hormones. Its contribution to my challenges was debated amongst doctors, and nothing else surfaced as an offending factor in our infertility. The reality is that 90% of infertility cases receive no answers. We were left to live with inconclusive results.

Instead of trying "a bunch more stuff," our reproductive endocrinologist (a mother of 10 children!) recommended moving to IVF. The intervention was out of alignment for me, way out of my comfort zone. Even so, I committed to giving it a try, knowing I could change my mind. A large brown box arrived in the mail, amber vials of viscous liquid surrounded by dry ice packs, pink, purple, and blue pills, soooo many needles. I wondered how people were allowed to do this to their own bodies at home. I shoved the box in the closet right away, out of sight, for three days and turned to prayer, breathwork, and meditation. In seeking the clarity to go for it, I got the "yes." I was 100 percent all-in on pursuing IVF as our path to parenthood.

Wouldn't you know, it worked. I got pregnant! My first pregnancy blessed me with twin boys. Bill and I walked around drunk with gratitude and delight. We were told we'd deliver early—twins and all—and as we rounded the corner towards the third trimester, I went into premature labor. They were born, stillborn, before we had the chance to meet them. Why wasn't my body able to do this? Wasn't I here to procreate? And if so, why was my equipment faulty? As I sifted through the torment and devastation of the loss, I found great solace in South American traditions. I readily embraced the idea that babies who "pass through" are sacred parts of our family, and we received glorious evidence to that end. On their due date, months after having delivered them, milk gushed spontaneously from my nipples. My breasts were geysers, affirming for me that I was still there for my twins, that I was a mother, still nourishing them. The milk felt like an offering, a ceremony of our unbounded connection. I called my gynecologist to ask her about the extraordinary event. She hurried to get off the phone without answering me about what was not found in Western medicine journals.

I was still broken, but the boys' ongoing presence vibrated around me. Our twins simply hold a different role in our family than they would if they were here in human form. We greet them on their birthday and wave at them from Earth.

I grieved, yet the life force within me screamed that I was still called to be a mother. In the ensuing years, I went through six more IVF cycles and the associated and countless pokes, prods, and procedures. I took Viagra suppositories (amazing for female libido, by the way), Lupron, Dexamethasone, learned the difference between subcutaneous and intramuscular injections, and shot my abdominal muscles and backsides full of enough hormones to affect a rhinoceros. We got pregnant again but miscarried early. Our savings dwindled to single digits, and I stopped answering the phone because every time someone called, it was to tell me they were pregnant again. My body and my spirit were frail, so a summertime visit from my parents was a welcome diversion. From the point of their arrival, my mother was jumpy and strange. Finally, she handed me a letter and explained that it contained an idea she had had. She strictly instructed me to read the letter in the other room and said we didn't ever have to speak of it again if I didn't want to. Likely, many of us have written in a letter a message we were too scared to deliver face-to-face. In this case, I believe Mom was scared I might perceive that she didn't believe in me or my abilities.

I myself no longer had faith in my body's ability to carry a child. I had surrendered our situation weeks prior to reading the letter. Bill and I wanted to be parents; we wanted to serve in that way. If it were meant to be, God would show us the way. Phrases from that letter swirl in my mind even now.

Postmenopausal women have given birth . . . I'm pretty good at this . . . Reason I have been able to get into great shape, have such great health . . . The happiest moments of my life were being pregnant and having you three girls.

Bill and I had been on such a strange journey, and the offer of my 61-year-old mother's surrogacy was even stranger. It was so bizarre, in fact, that I knew immediately that it was the way we would become parents. An electric sensation pulsed through me, and I knew with certainty and on a very deep level that this offer was divinely guided. There are so many miraculous details about how I experienced the pregnancy alongside my mom (attending every appointment, sharing every joy and every concern), how she made headlines as one of the oldest women ever to give birth, and the remarkable gift she gave us in Finn, Bill's and my biological son. It's a story in and of itself. But right now, I'm here to acknowledge in a transparent, real, non-fairytale sort of way a few of my experiences as a new mother. I hope they normalize some of the experiences you're having or may have had, whether you had a traditional pregnancy or something far more out there like I did.

My parents stayed with us for the first two weeks following Finn's arrival before returning home. We had lived in our little pod for months, and it was time for them to start the next chapter of their own lives. My mom is often asked whether leaving us (namely Finn) was difficult. Her response is always quick, "No, I never wanted to be a parent again. I was super excited to be a grandmother." Fortunately, we didn't have any pain around that. She was always energetically clear on Finn being her grandchild. "He's just sleeping in your old room," she'd joke, referring to her uterus. My mother's departure cued my moment to step into motherhood . . . fully. My copilot was gone. It was all me.

Have I earned the honor of motherhood? Am I doing this right? Is my body defective? Am I dedicated enough to motherhood amongst my myriad other responsibilities? Amid the euphoria brought on by finally (oh my gosh it's really real) having a healthy, alive child, these imposter questions swirled in my brain.

I had planned to take a four to six month leave from my coaching career and writing. I wanted to savor the blessed opportunity I had to be a mother. Bill's role as the breadwinner, along with his total support of me as a mother, allowed me the luxury of being fully present with Finn. He and I were closely bonded from the moment he was placed in my arms, perhaps underwritten by our biological connection and the privilege of having lived the pregnancy with my mother. He had heard my voice every night as I read Harry Potter and poured my love through my mother's belly. Mothers who don't carry their babies worry about this; we were very fortunate. Ecstasy oozed from my every cell. Dreams really do come true! I pinched myself, unable to fully believe that he was here.

I answered Finn's cries with joy and so much enthusiasm to right his every woe. I know it sounds disingenuous, but I'm being serious. I knew what it was like to come home to an empty nursery, and I knew I would never take my alive baby for granted. Paranoia poked temporary holes in the elation, however, as historical trauma led to hypervigilance and co-sleeping. I needed instant confirmation that he was breathing. I met with a therapist who told me I needed to stop checking on him so many times throughout the night. Fat chance, I thought. I worked through the anxiety and slowly took the air out of the PTSD balloon a little at a time. I did the therapy to be able to inherently trust that because he'd made it here, he would stay here, stay alive.

I was excited to experience all aspects of new motherhood. While Mom was still pregnant, I met with a functional medicine doctor who told me how I might be able to bring in milk again through herbs, visualizations, and pumping. I knew it wasn't a sure thing, but it felt like a cool thing to try. Finn was so eager and skilled at latching that he earned himself the nickname of "little shark." Because my body produced only a meager amount of milk, I taped an SNS (Supplemental Nursing System) tube to my nipple, and he received formula in addition to my milk. I nursed a couple times a day and bottle-fed him otherwise. I was so extremely clear on how lucky I was to be a mother that I couldn't let how I fed Finn mean something.

I was successful at not obsessing about the matter until I showed up with a friend to a local La Leche League meeting. She told me how welcoming the group was and how much the community helped her with her first baby. Dizzy with excitement to finally be on the inside of this club and eager for the camaraderie of the new community, I mingled with the other mothers. As the official meeting commenced, the tone changed as woman after woman spoke about the essentiality of breastfeeding. One woman said she'd read a study where mothers who didn't breastfeed raised serial killers. The message was clear: if you don't breastfeed, you're a monster. Not only a horrible mother, but a horrible person.

I sat numb and felt shame rise from my feet like a fire. I wondered if any of these women had lost a child, suffered a miscarriage, or endured a stillbirth. Because if so, I couldn't imagine they would be so quick to demonize women who were doing their best with what we had. I slinked out to sob in my car. I sobbed because I was ostracized by a group I had hoped would welcome and support me. In my first attempt at community in motherhood, I was shunned for not being able to execute one aspect of the job in one particular way.

I shook off the meeting and focused on the miracle strapped to my chest by a cotton sling. I reminded myself that I believe in soul contracts. I believe that Finn chose me as his mother. He chose the way he came into this world, and he chose me with this body ... and what it can and cannot do. That, coupled with my boundless joy in being a mother, allowed me to let go of a convention that didn't work for me (us). I look back with fondness at the 10 weeks Finn was at my breast, and I hold no regrets about my decision to fully bottle feed him after that. My only regret is how I shamed myself in response to how women treated other women at a time when walls needed to be dismantled, not further cemented. At a time when altruistic, non-judgmental support would go such a long way.

While scarred from the experience, those women at the meeting couldn't keep me down. My rapture with Finn continued with every day we spent together. Professor Dumbledore gifted Harry Potter an invisibility cloak left to him by his late father, providing keen coverage and protection against his nemeses. I felt myself wrapped in a gratitude cloak endowed to me by the infertility fairies. My deep and active gratitude freed me from some of the typical expressions of shock around the radical drop into new motherhood. "Holy cow, this is so hard" and "OMG, the sleepless nights suck" weren't vernacular in my head or out of my mouth. I felt anxious at night and disoriented from lack of sleep, but the undercurrent from my long, rough, and extreme path to motherhood blessed me with a superpower. I lived to choose Finn's daily outfit (Baby jeans! Infant fisherman sweaters!) and set the route for our long strolls. My cloak wasn't completely impermeable, however. The sleep deprivation eventually caught up to me. Bill and I had decided that while I was on maternity leave and he was working, I would command the night shift. We had an agreement, and I did my part happily. Until, for the first time in the nine years we had been together, I sat on resentment that bubbled up from dark, dank places. I noticed myself scorekeeping the way I'd seen other women do but I'd never done.

He's had a solid seven hours of sleep, I thought, watching Bill waltz over to pick up Finn. It must be nice.

"So, we're keeping score now," Bill asked, fiery, after I finally verbalized my disdain. "You think I do nothing?"

"It's not like that," I said. But it was like that. "It just seems like your life hasn't changed much, and I'm up every night in a Groundhog Day loop."

That was the first of several prickly illustrations of a new dynamic that had crept into our marriage. My new variety of annoyance toward Bill startled me, and I didn't like it. I started adding up how many diapers I'd changed, how many loads and unloads of the dishwasher, the laundry. He looked stung when I whined about these things, and he actually was doing quite a bit.

"I'm not one of those guys," he said, referring to friends of ours who participated in childrearing like it was the 1950s. "I'm all-in on this with you."

Luckily, I had done a lot of personal growth work in my 20s, so I was able to quickly name the scorekeeping and shift it before it became too toxic. We discussed what we could do differently and how I could get my needs met. I hadn't asked for more help. I had expected him to read my mind. The conversations were raw and revealed things to and about both of us. I was happy to do the bulk of the baby tasks. I wanted to. But I also wanted more care, more acknowledgment, more SLEEP. Following a few bouts of raised voices and tears, we were reminded that we're stronger together, and we recommitted to airing even—especially—what felt like the small stuff.

About 12 weeks into loving on Finn, I started to crave balance earlier than expected. Our days were repetitive, and I desired stimulation that was something other than baby care. My work has always been a calling; it's not just a job to me. I didn't dwell on why the need for balance came up earlier than expected, and I opened my mind and heart back to my work and eased into reconnecting with three clients. As soon as I did, another thing happened. I got a book deal. Remember I said our surrogacy journey was a story? Well, I meant that, literally. In addition to my work as a coach, I'm a writer. In the years leading up to Finn, I struggled not only at fertility but also at captivating publishers with my various manuscripts. They claimed to like my writing but didn't believe I had written the right book . . . yet.

When Mom was six months pregnant, and with her generous support and that of my father and Bill (since it was their story, too), I contacted my literary agent and imparted our extraordinary story. She flipped, in the best sense, and promised to start pitching it to publishers. My dream of writing and actually publishing a book was rekindled. My agent instructed me to journal every day to capture every pertinent detail of the tale. I felt the new promise of an eventual book, but I didn't journal. I couldn't. All the dreadful memories of loss flooded back. Call it superstitious, or call it self-protection, but I feared that writing down what was going so well might risk a good outcome.

As life would have it, my two big dreams converged upon

each other and happened at once. A baby and a book! Suddenly and urgently, I had to redesign my time. One of these initiatives alone would have kept me busy. I was behind before I even started because I hadn't followed the suggestion to journal in the back-third of Mom's pregnancy and in the first three months of Finn's life. No stranger to deadlines, I leaped to a rigid writing schedule supportive of big deliverables. I wrote pretty much whenever Finn slept, day and night. My mind was a fountain, recalling all the details that I hadn't written down. I discovered ways to hold Finn and type at the same time, and I honored my client commitments. There weren't enough hours in the day. Finn came first, then the book, then Bill. At some point, my duo of dreams started to duel. Were they actually dueling, or was I just not adequate? I fought through waves of guilt. I was finally a mother. Shouldn't I devote every second to our baby after what we'd been through? I would find a way to balance better. It was all almost too good to be true, and I couldn't let any of it slip through my fingers.

I was fortunate to find a local graduate student to come to the house and care for Finn as I wrote feverishly in the next room. Pages were being produced, and I could see for myself that Finn was in excellent hands. As soon as I let myself feel excited about finally having a legit book deal, I was overcome with insidious guilt over diverting any iota of my attention away from Finn. I'd waited this long to have a baby, and now I was going to hand him over to someone else. My acute discomfort at that juncture was around my soul's knowing that I'm on this earth to fulfill things in addition to being a mother. The problem was that I was bucking up against another conditioned expectation of what it meant to be a good mother. I'd finally eked out self-permission to work and parent simultaneously and was feeling good about my decisions, but I'd held onto another insidious belief: that in order to be a good mother, I would have no needs of my own and no agenda other than caring for and serving my child. I should have no time for myself or for my own dreams. This was modeled to me by my own loving mother, who set herself aside to raise me and my sisters. It was modeled to me by other family members and by friends and acquaintances who chose stay-at-home motherhood over working motherhood.

One afternoon, I finished my writing early. Our sitter was still scheduled to care for Finn for several hours. Spontaneously, primally even, I acted on a desire that had been continuously popping into my mind. How lavish it would be to sit by myself in a cool theater and watch a movie. For six months, I had done nothing other than care for Finn and do my work, my only two self-permitted activities. Despite being magnetically drawn to the big screen, my body quivered as I sat, and I couldn't settle in my seat. What was I doing alone in a dark space away from my baby? I was a horrible person. As the previews rolled and the main attraction began, I wrapped myself tight in my sweater and my mind slowly left my head. For two hours, I escaped to the heartwarming story (resplendently possessing no parallels to my own life) and its well-developed characters. I laughed, and I cried. My initial physical and emotional discomfort transformed into a state of overflowing hope and opportunity.

Who says mothers can't do anything for ourselves? Who dictates that we can't have a break? Who orders us to deplete ourselves in service to another, or others? *Who says?* By the time I got home, I had birthed a new paradigm, one according to which *I* would determine what it meant to be a good mother. I received downloads from the Universe and was laser clear on what would fill me up, what would allow me to be the very best mother to Finn and the best wife to Bill. I had a new plan. In addition to mothering and meeting my publisher's deadlines, I would go to yoga once a week, see a friend for lunch, or go to an art museum. I committed to filling myself personally and professionally so that I could best fill others. When *Bringing in Finn* came out, I knew I'd honored all of me and our family, and I had modeled for others.

Society sentimentalizes motherhood. I see culture fetishizing a joyful pregnancy and a fantastical newborn phase. It's all true and also not true. The bliss and the ecstasy are surely there, but so too are shock, overwhelm, unworthiness, and so many other emotions. My fertility story ended well, fairytale well. While our real-life experiences and relationships often don't mimic those of published fairytales, we can write our own happy endings. Dreams do come true! Keep dreaming, keep trusting, and keep trying however you know how. Don't concern yourself with how your life looks compared to those of others. Your life is as it is because it's meant for you and no one else. Hold it tight; it's yours. It's your precious, perfect gift. Do it your way.

Know thyself and to thine own self be true. The more I've been able to trust and live by that mantra—instead of grappling with fulfilling an ideal that's been imposed on me—the more I like how I show up as a mother. I'm not perfect; I slip up all the time. But I'm honest about it: I own it, and I'm open to discussion about it. Your child chose you, and you chose your child. You are meant to be together, just as you are. To all mothers, no matter how your baby came into your arms, I wish you trust in your unique, beautiful, divinely intended way of becoming—and being—a mother.

Chapter 6

Amazing Grace

SHERYL

* * *

"Not flesh of my flesh, nor bone of my bone,
but still miraculously my own.
Never forget for a single minute
that you didn't grow under my heart, but in it."

—Fleur Conkling Heyliger

I suppose you could say I've always been comfortable speaking my mind. Over the years—and across professions—I've used my understanding and extrapolation of the facts to thoughtfully affect outcomes. My earliest memory of such efforts was a multi-installment plea to my mother for a baby sister. For context, *Parent Trap* was a hot film at the time and likely inspired my specific desire for a twin sister. I was old enough to loosely understand the impossibility of that happening, so I set my sights on becoming a big sister. My older brother was pretty cool and served his purpose just fine, but I desperately wanted a baby in the family. I wrote persuasive letters and held family meetings at the dinner table. I intuitively knew to target my mother with my modest request.

Early responses weren't encouraging, so I pressed harder and identified what I believed to be brilliant rebuttals to each rejection I encountered. To her justification of being too old, I researched how mature women could manage to have babies and countered with the option of adoption. Our family didn't have copious material possessions, but we had abundant love. Surely, we could accommodate just one more child. Despite my best and heartfelt efforts, I didn't win the battle.

My parents were very loving, and they did their best for us in every capacity. Mom was an only child and always lamented that, often speaking of her childhood loneliness. Her mother died young, leaving Mom to singlehandedly manage the health issues of her father. It was again lonely. My mother leaned on me heavily. More than that even, she lived through my brother and me. By the time I was a teen, I could appreciate the backdrop of the situation. Mom had finished her coursework for a Master's thesis in social work at the University of Chicago but never completed it. The explanation included that she met and married my father, and they thought WWII was going to take him overseas. At the war's conclusion, they started a family, and she never made it back to her schooling. As a young person, I had the calamity of her unfulfilled personal goal emblazoned in my mind. Further, it became clear to me that her intense focus on how my brother and I achieved, and the importance she assigned to our accomplishments, directly resulted from her inability to achieve her own goal. Her living through us had real implications for how we both responded and the pressures we felt.

At times, growing up, I had difficulty separating my identity from that of my mother. Did I like the dress, or did she? Did I study my tail off and get the A+ for my own reward or for hers? She was a very dutiful and doting mother, but on the same token, I had a challenge separating, and that felt like a pressure. Earlier than I could put my finger on the psychology and pathology at hand, I knew it felt bad, and I committed two things to myself: #1 I wouldn't lose myself in marriage or motherhood, and #2 I wouldn't inflict the same co-dependent pressures on my own child(ren) one day. I would give them ample opportunities to discover their own calling and joy. I'll call these my "SCs," my self-commitments.

I was blessed with a good brain as the foundation of my young academic prowess, and I paired that potential with both intrinsic and extrinsic motivation. I can say with much gratitude that things worked out for me. I excelled through high school, undergraduate collegiate education, law school, and additional post-graduate degrees. My early career was augmented with hobbies and a courtship and eventual marriage to Charlie. Everything was proceeding according to my liking (and my mother's satisfaction) until I made some headlines that were very different from the ones about which I'd dreamt.

One of my aforementioned hobbies was learning to fly. My need for speed and efficiency in life translated well to the cockpit, and so I was invigorated behind the wheel in the sky. The story of my first solo flight at the age of 29 was one of engine failure and inferno. By the grace of God, I was able to land the plane without harming others, but the fiery crash did a doozy on me. Burned across 37% of my body and given a 10% chance of survival following one of seven major surgeries, I spent two months in the hospital and returned there every day for two years for rehabilitation therapy.

A lot about the crash was fateful, including the fact that I lived, period. Remember my two SCs? Well, my crash and ensuing recovery period spurred a third SC: #3 I would challenge the maxim of "everything in moderation." That's right. I would do exactly nothing in moderation, and this meant asserting myself fully when justice was on the line, breaking glass ceilings, and loving those who needed it the most . . . because tomorrow is not guaranteed. Another result of the crash and my significant injuries was our decision about how to become parents.

Following a period of literally getting back on my feet and a slow transition of my days away from the burn clinic and occupational therapy and back to work, I recall thinking it was time to get back on track with starting our family. Charlie and I had been married for three years at that point. Prior to the crash, we had envisioned and spoken in unrestrained, dreamy hypotheticals about a family: the footsteps of a deftly curious boy and a tenderly poised girl, born at least two years apart and fast friends.

The drastic disruption of the crash and my long recovery materially changed our conversations about parenthood. Without rattling off all the details, one significant complication I experienced was a burst intestine, which required an ileostomy. While I wasn't told by the doctors that I wouldn't be able to have biological children, my body was wrecked. I had the help of renowned medical professionals and an immense organic drive to build myself back up, yet I was significantly damaged and recognized my physical limitations. Everything hurt. Dealing with all that we had, adoption came to us quickly as a stellar way to move forward with our plans to parent. Neither a stated necessity nor a last resort, the adoption option seemed highly reasonable given the circumstances.

Adoption wasn't foreign to us. Please recall that I used it as the premise of those early persuasive speeches to my mother. We also had family friends who had adopted four children, all of whom were in our wedding party. I saw the love in their family, and I construed their family unit to be something very special, in no way compromised by the absence of genetics or the birth process for my friend. As soon as I could think beyond my own medical needs, we applied to two adoption agencies: Children's Home Society of Minnesota and Lutheran Social Services.

They were the largest and most familiar to me, so that's where we started.

Ours was a careful and thoughtful plan. It was our Plan A. It was not Plan B for us, which it seems many assume adoption is for parents. Through lengthy discussions, we wrestled with our souls in terms of what we could see ourselves doing as adoptive parents. Could we handle a child with a physical disability? If so, what kind? Could we support a child with mental or emotional issues? Were we willing to consider Fetal Alcohol Syndrome babies? To me, these questions and their answers position adoption as a truly intentional form of parenting. When one conceives and carries her biological child, choices exist along the way for insight into her fetus's health condition. Examples include ultrasound imaging, blood-based genetic testing, amniocentesis, etc. Depending on what's learned, there are choices that follow for some.

We had to think even more in advance about what our capabilities, interests, strengths, and weaknesses might be as parents. One of the questions was whether we would consider a foreign-born child. That one wasn't a hard one for us. We knew quickly that we would consider a baby from another country. There were Korean children in Minnesota. In fact, at the time, the state had the largest population of Korean-born children due specifically to the Children's Home Society and a Korean social worker on staff there. My father was the only individual in the mix who had an issue with this. He challenged us point blank and couldn't understand why we couldn't find a Caucasian child. I felt strongly that what we were doing was the right thing, so my father's negativity didn't influence me. Instead, I tried hard to understand his lens and focused on helping him adjust. To his dying day, he denied his skepticism (alright, outright unacceptance) around a Korean baby because he had such a beautiful and strong relationship with our daughter.

Unlike a pregnancy's progressive parameter of nine months, we had been in a holding pattern for two whole years. We had prepared the nursery and shopped for clothing and accessories. That was the same as a biological path to parenthood, but in addition to those preparations, we really wanted to delve into the cultural piece. How were we going to handle a child of a different culture? I'll discuss later some of our related choices when she was a bit older, but there were cultural matters of consideration even in infancy. The agency was excellent at preparing us and facilitating groups of other couples awaiting Korean babies. We covered the same topics as most expectant parent classes: feeding, diapering, sleeping, bathing, etc. But we also talked about the medical side of things, including the fact that most Korean babies are born with a milk intolerance. That meant we fed her a special variety of Similac formula. The community was wonderfully helpful and supportive, and we developed deep and lasting connections with our peers.

We knew we would receive a girl due to availability. Boys weren't available because they're valued in Korean culture. Girls, however, didn't have a real identity, especially if they were illegitimate. After the interminably long years of waiting, we got the call, "the referral." Eun Joo Yoon, a baby girl, was available, and we would call her Sarah. We had known for a while that her name would be Sarah, after my paternal grandmother, and we would use her family name of Yoon as her middle name. We could have waited even longer for a Caucasian baby, but it didn't dawn on us to go that route because we were entirely comfortable adopting Sarah. We were told she could be with us in just three or four days!

I've been asked when I first felt like a mother, identified as a mother. That's easy: when we received the photo as part of the referral and named her. That's when Sarah was ours; that was the moment of imprint for me. Through the photographic paper, her eyes pierced mine, and they captured my heart. I would liken it to what I've heard is the experience of seeing an early ultrasound image of one's biological baby in-utero. That photo is in her baby book and comes to mind effortlessly. She needed me, and I needed her. It was pretty much that simple and that profound. That's why, when we received a call the next day that there may be a glitch, it was so very painful. The Korean agency explained that there was concern about Sarah's eyes and her premature birth, indicating there might be an anomaly with her brain's development. Knowing what to do, how to proceed, was difficult and confusing. She was in Korea; we were here. The quality of medical care available there was unclear and concerned us. We couldn't facilitate our own assessment, and more importantly, we were already in love. In another fateful occurrence, there happened to be a group of American military doctors on-site at the agency at that exact time. The group included a pediatrician, and they agreed to look at Sarah.

While we awaited their report, we were again placed on emotional hold as to whether she would be coming to live with us in three short days. I will never forget the next call. The doctor had said to the agency liaison, "Congratulate the parents. She's the cutest, smartest little girl we've ever seen, and they're very lucky to be her parents." Her parents! I set out to purchase announcements and invitations but didn't end up having enough time to get them out. Her plane arrived 36 hours later. We had waited two years, but somehow, it still felt sudden.

Our arrival day was different from many. Sarah's homecoming looked like 40 people at the airport gate greeting her with balloons, open arms, and endless love. That's how we received Sarah, how she was "born" to us. I stood expectantly at the front of our welcoming party with my eyes fixed tightly on every disembarking passenger. My heart fluttered intermittently. Finally, about 10 minutes into the exodus, I saw a perfectly demure woman carrying an infant sized about right. As I met her eyes, mine filled with tears. We nodded simultaneously as she continued her approach, and the escort handed me my firstborn child. I didn't feel like I was meeting Sarah for the first time. But the tactile details of her scent, her soft cheek against mine, and how her head fit perfectly between my chin and neck were glorious new inputs to my nervous system. They screamed motherhood.

It was not the same as a mucus-covered baby, still attached by an umbilical cord, being handed to its mother by an obstetrician. But it was just as special, just as sweet. It was not a diminished delivery experience in the least bit. My deep desire for motherhood came true that day, and our joint journey as mother and daughter began. Well after the jet bridge door had closed, and following an extended period of oohing, aahing and passing Sarah around the gallery, we moved the masses to our house to celebrate. One perk of adoption is that one isn't postpartum in a physical sense. Hormones don't rage, and your body is intact (barring any pre-existing conditions, including plane crashes). In fact, I experienced such a high from the time we received the referral call that I pulled off some really fine party details if I do say so myself. For those old enough to remember Northwest Airlines, we had a cake shaped like the plane that delivered Sarah to us. While my emotions were too frenetic (in a good way) on Sarah's arrival day to realize it then, it's not lost on me that a two-seater Piper Tomahawk aircraft robbed me of a lot, nearly my life, and a massive Boeing 777 delivered my baby, made me a mother.

A whole new world began. There was no warmup lap; the sprint began immediately. I was ready to take on my new role and the new title of mother/Mom. As timing would have it, I had acquired another new role and the title of judge/Your Honor only five weeks prior. A lot was happening all at once, and Sarah's arrival day was the only day I took off from work. I was back on the bench the next day. I asked my colleague and close friend if he wanted to come home with me at lunch to meet my new baby, and there commenced my juggling act. At that time, there wasn't an emphasis on maternity leave. Professional women did it all without ample recognition... and way ahead of current-day discussions of work-life balance and self-care.

Although I didn't pause per se, nurturing the precious, new little person in my life came naturally and easily as after-hours work. I was, in essence, an around-the-clock worker before receiving Sarah, and I didn't immediately change the number of hours I worked or the rigor of that work. But I adjusted and reallocated. As I approached any new role, I practiced patience with all involved and dove from the high dive into the deep end. I formed and led a team around me to help care for Sarah. I was extremely fortunate to have parents who were able and willing to spend a lot of time with her while I lined up a nanny. An at-home care arrangement and a close relationship with that individual were highly important to us. We were blessed to find Anita, who quickly became another member of our family. The relationship between Anita and Sarah was so close that Anita ended up naming her first child Sarah. She and Charlie were my co-pilots, if you will, and we shared the flight well.

Most of my friends were co-workers, and we didn't socialize as families. My brother didn't have children yet, so I really hadn't been exposed to babies. I never babysat and hadn't changed a diaper or held a bottle. I was totally inexperienced. Being a rule follower myself, in addition to one who enforced the rules in the courtroom, I attempted to adhere to the three-page summary provided to us about how to feed Sarah. It was the closest thing to an instruction manual I expect ever comes with a baby. But the reality was that we would form a new routine, one suited to the two of us. I gave us grace in developing that routine, and it wasn't always pretty trying to sync her needs and my schedule.

To boot, two weeks after getting Sarah, I had subsequent surgery on my right hand, the one that had been burnt to the bone. So, I wasn't even able to change her diaper for a while. But we got by, and those early weeks represented life-long bonding between us.

I didn't ever stop working professionally, but I did constantly strive for balance and found creative ways to combine mothering and a demanding career. Most weeknights, I was home around dinner time and was able to feed and bathe Sarah myself. My workdays often flew by in anticipation of our evenings together. Even if I missed dinner, I was always home to rock her to sleep singing "Amazing Grace." That time together, snuggling in the rocker was sacred. It was the climax of individual days and a validation that we were meant to be together in this life. On weekends I tried to devote the majority of my time to her. If I had to work, I would do so at home with her.

Continuing and advancing my career was my ticket to not letting happen to me what happened to my mother (living with an unfulfilled goal). It's how I fulfilled SC #1: not losing myself within marriage or motherhood. I didn't feel that my professional success was a slight to my children. On the contrary, I was a better mother to them because I kept myself whole. No one else was going to do that for me, so I did it for myself. I want to be clear about for whom I worked. I did my work for me and for my new family. Sure, I trust and hope my accomplishments pleased my mother along the way, but I did the work for my own sake.

Likewise, my career was part of how I wouldn't do to my daughter what my mother did to me (living vicariously through me and imposing, at times, stifling pressure). If I was fulfilled personally, then I could properly foster Sarah's unique identity and pursuits. SC #2: supporting my children in finding their own purpose and pleasure in life.

My challenge was to be aggressive professionally while at the same time being there as Sarah's mother. I had pondered this challenge quite carefully before receiving her. I had a plan, and I was up for it. But when she arrived, the fear factor set in. The fear was real and went beyond conscious calculation. At times, it felt like panic, and logic wasn't a reliable antidote. Some new mothers obsess over how much their babies eat or sleep or how all the soiled laundry will get done. I figured those details would work themselves out. My daydreams and nightmares focused on how I would avoid living my life through her without putting up walls and creating unhealthy distance, for the sake of both of us. My approach to parenting was highly conscientious, maybe too much so. It certainly wasn't lighthearted, but it was absolutely full of tremendous heart. It was time to walk the talk, time to turn my self-commitments into reality.

From day one, I have been very respectful of my daughter as a separate person with her own life. I wanted to see her as a different person from myself. On the surface, literally on our skin's surface, we didn't match. And I liked that. I didn't want us to be one and the same, and my intention was for her to eventually feel that herself. I wanted to expose Sarah to as much as possible and to opportunities that I myself didn't have. So, I blocked my work schedule, and Anita would bring Sarah to me at lunchtime so we could attend Music for the Very Young and swimming classes together when she was just six months old. As she got a little older, I didn't miss one special event at daycare. I have the funniest and most precious memory of a Suzuki piano recital when she was two years old. Her performance entailed bowing only, as it was all she could manage at the time. My hope, mindset, and genuine intention was to give her myriad opportunities (not only those I assumed she'd be interested in) from which to craft her own tapestry of talents, interests, and choices.

As mentioned earlier, we never lost sight of the cultural piece for Sarah. It was our job to make the adjustments, not hers. She hadn't asked to be here; that was our idea. We constantly asked ourselves how we would ensure that she didn't feel like a stranger in a strange land among Caucasian parents and grandparents, a white neighborhood, and white classmates. Eventually, we chose private schooling for her, as there was more cultural diversity in the private sector where we lived than in the public sector.

After finding our groove the best we could as parents, Charlie and I went on to adopt two more children. I wholeheartedly believe that parenting via adoption is in no way a lesser method of becoming a parent. But I guess I can't be the judge of that since I don't know what I missed by not carrying and birthing a biological child. I can't issue a factual statement, only an opinion based on my own experience. I believe that parenting through adoption may be an even greater method. I have found it to be most intentional: the timing is intentional, and the criteria around what type of child you will be a parent of are intentional. Adoption is not the opportunity to have a perfect or rosy family. Rather, it's the call to give love, mercy, and patience.

Our second child, Charlie, is Caucasian, and our third, Kristina, is Korean. Despite our thinking that we were most likely done after two, Sarah tugged at our hearts at the age of five when she asked for a baby sister. Perhaps she had success where I hadn't at a similar age because she had a significantly more persuasive, emotional, and actionable plea. She instinctively commented that when Charlie got older, he would look like Charlie and me, but she wouldn't. "I really would like a little sister," Sarah said. Enough said. We were sold. Sarah would win the battle I had lost all those years back, and that's when we put in the application to adopt Kristina. We came to the top of the list as soon as we got Sarah. That meant the agency would have secured us a baby the following week, but we weren't ready. We were at the top of the Caucasian list at that point as well, but we wanted to meet Sarah's criterion (and our own) for our third child . . . a

Korean girl. Sarah took Kristina to "Sharing Day" in kindergarten class that year. I don't think life gets much better.

It happens often that people ask if Charlie is our "own" because of his race. Correcting this inquiry has always poked my propensity to speak my mind, and I always respond joyfully with "They are ALL our OWN children." I find the rest to be none of their business. I have also been asked if upon determining our desire for additional children, we ever considered trying for biological children since I was further recovered at that point. The answer is no. Even if we could have had biological children, we knew that adoption was right for us. Our family portrait of one Caucasian female, two Caucasian males, and two Korean females is picture-perfect. And I will be the judge of that!

Our babies' arrival days were life-altering days for us, and we celebrate the dates every year. When they were school-aged, we would bring Korean pear apples that day or read Korean fairy tales. I brought treat bags of decorated rice crispy treats for each child in Charlie's class. One of Sarah's classmates once said she wished she were adopted so she, too, could celebrate two "birthdays" each year. Once again, adoption looked like an optimal choice . . . two celebrations a year! I wanted them to feel proud that those who had given birth to them couldn't provide for them but loved them so much that they arranged for them to come live with us.

SC #3 is a summative one. My mission to do nothing in moderation impacts all aspects of my life and those who share it. I continued my trajectory in the legal field and became involved in causes that inspired me. Bicycle rides with the kids were a must, and birthday parties and Halloween costume parties were elaborate events. So, what gave? There were tolls along the way, things like lost sleep and chronic bronchitis. But I managed and never felt like the balance wasn't working for me or for Sarah. We checked in with each other on that often. I tried to give all that I could to both my professional life and motherhood, and I tried hard to never deprive Sarah of my fullest attention.

Although it wasn't my goal, I eventually felt good about and believed in the headlines I made. I was featured as a woman to watch. The details of my plane crash, family built through adoption, senior titles in law (federal prosecutor, public defender, judge, Commissioner of Corrections) and nursing (doctorate of nursing practice), significant volunteer work (general counsel to Children's Home Society) and completed marathons (seven) were highlighted in local and national newspapers and magazines. They said I was a trailblazer who was doing it all. I didn't see myself as such, but rather as someone doing the best I could for myself, my children, my husband, my clients, my courtroom, and my patients. I am ongoingly focused on giving back to the organizations that gave me my family and lending hope to fellow burn victims. I held onto my personal identity and, therefore, was able to raise my children to be soulful people with their own identities. I could have done without the press coverage, but I was happy if my story could help or inspire others.

I expect most people have "things" with which they had issue relative to their own upbringing. I bet many even hold fear like mine of being like their parents. Whatever your personal fears might be, each is legitimate and worthy of recognition. Use your fear to inspire action. As I've shared, I translated my fears into a living mantra: my three SCs. I'm proud that my new motherhood experience with Sarah was riddled with fear and anxiety about parenting her differently than I was parented. It was scary and at times, downright terrifying. But because I confronted the fear head-on, today I believe that women can effectively embody both identities: professional and mother. Oh, and throw in spouse, if that's you. When the string ensemble at Sarah's wedding played "Amazing Grace" and I heard her singing it to her own babies at bedtime, I knew our evenings were sacred to her as well.

I gave my mother grace; she did her very, very best for us. I gave myself grace; I wasn't a perfect mother, and I wasn't a perfect judge. I gave Sarah grace; she landed here from a land far, far away. I gave everyone around us grace, and it served us well. Please give yourself lots and lots of grace right now, no matter where you are on your mothering journey. Give yourself enough respect and grace to identify your very own SCs. They will become your pillars for motherhood and for life. You are amazing.

Chapter 7

The Married Single Mom

BRIE

> *"At times in life we feel lost or strange, even in crowds of people we know. But once in a while we meet someone, and our heart says, 'Oh, there you are. I've been looking for you.' Eventually, we find our tribe."*
>
> —Unknown

In a perilous move, I transferred Matty from a sound sleep in the swing to the car seat carrier. By some miracle, I managed to secure the harness, exit the condo, enter the garage, and snap the carrier into the car's base without him waking up. I took that accomplishment in and of itself to be the Universe urging me to make this departure happen.

After finally fastening my own seat belt, I caught the clock out of the corner of my eye. 10:16 am, 11 minutes late. The defeat stung, and so did my hand from the blow to the steering wheel. First impressions were my thing, or at least they always had been. I'd wanted to arrive at the hospital early, so I could be composed and pleasant meeting the other ladies at the postpartum group. Via Lake Shore Drive and with minimal traffic, the jaunt from Lakeview to Chicago's Gold Coast was a good 20 minutes. There was no way I'd make the 10:30 am start, not unless LSD were sprinkled with fairy speed dust.

My heart raced, but the rest of me was paralyzed. It was no flippant excursion. Meticulous preparations began the night before, and I'd been pondering the sequence of the morning for days. I reviewed the registration email and start time. I set multiple alarms just in case I actually slept. I packed and re-packed every compartment of the diaper bag and made a list of questions. I even showered and put on mascara—big accomplishments.

It was decision time, and I couldn't let all that work go to waste. Heck, I was dressed in something other than yoga pants. My contacts felt like shards of glass in my eyes since I hadn't needed those alarms after all. We were out of the house. I repeat, we were out of the house! I contemplated driving around the block and going right back to the condo. Javi was out the door early for the office, so he never would have known of my massive failure. But he'd been so encouraging about going to the group, and I didn't want to let him down.

You have to do something! At least pull out of the garage, you coward.

It was the first time I was driving solo with Matty, our maiden voyage. I craned my neck to check on him in the "rear-view mirror" hanging from the captain seat's headrest and cheered myself on. *I've got this. I have to do this. I must re-enter the world.* It was time. I told myself that if the group was horrible, I didn't need to go back the following week. My heart was still racing, and I relied on muscle memory as I pulled out of the garage and turned left out of the alley. My OB's office was adjacent to the hospital, so I knew the route well. Matty was gloriously quiet. *I can do this.*

We hit all the red lights, which gave me time to dig a tube of lip gloss out of the car-door pocket and find my words for when I was asked how we were doing. I envisioned the introduction of mothers and babies, and with everything else to prepare, I hadn't refined that "elevator speech." I'd struggled for the eight weeks since Matty had been born, and I didn't know how to admit it in a respectable way. I knew to expect up to seven other new mothers, and I had a mental image of who they would be. Book club types. They'd have their acts together. They'd be adept at nursing in public, stylish cover and all. Unlike me, they'd be fully immersed in their new identities as mothers and accepting of the lives they had left behind. I doubted very much that any one of them could have been having as hard a time as me. The monotony, the sleepless day-night cycles, and the challenge of keeping both of us clean had landed me in a deep hole. I reminded myself that I didn't have to say anything I didn't want to. I could just listen.

By no surprise, we were late. I'd made up some time in the left lane, but it was still 10:35 am before I saw the big blue "H" sign at our exit. It was mid-morning for crying out loud. I had never been late for work or a meeting; now, rush hour was over, and I still couldn't get there on time.

Feeling nauseous and as if my heart might finally beat out of my chest, I pulled into the valet circle drive of Northwestern's Prentice Women's Hospital. With shaky, sweaty hands, I stopped and ejected Matty's carrier. Maybe I was shaky from the caffeine I was not so effectively avoiding, or maybe it was just nerves. The blended scents of antiseptic and floral notes inspired nostalgia as the double glass doors slid open. It was my first return to the hospital since delivering Matty. On no previous occasion would I have required valet parking service, a volunteer escort, or even signage to find the red pin on the directory's map. Room 112-C was located just down the hallway from the bustling lobby. The adrenaline of the drive wore off quickly, and the mental and physical tolls of the past 16 hours—actually the past eight weeks—set in. I was in a haze and politely accepted the aproned volunteer's offer to chaperone me to the classroom, aware of the pity he must have felt for me. The carrier cut deeper and deeper into the inside of my forearm as we walked (because, notwithstanding my checklist, I had forgotten the portable stroller base). My sheer top was soaked with more than a glistening; I think even my toenails were sweating at that point.

The last time I was in the building, I radiated the expectant bliss of bringing new life into the world. This time, I was panicked and sullen. The chasm between expectation and reality in this life event was wide. I digress. One thing was the same, though; I was wearing the same pair of maternity jeans I'd worn the day Matty was born. I'd gone from wanting to model my beautiful belly to wanting to hide the aftermath. My choice of tunic nicely disguised the elastic waistband and muffin top. I could only hope that the suede booties distracted from the wet circles under my arms and supported the appearance of a moderately fashion-conscious, self-respecting individual.

When we arrived at the room, I peered in from the safety of the doorway. The u-shaped configuration of tables and chairs was residual of the conference room's last occupants, perhaps an administrative team in suits and heels or a group of department chiefs between surgeries collaborating to solve the woes of healthcare in this country. I absorbed the ambiance, which was anything but sterile. It was reassuringly calm, actually, apart from a muffled fuss and one mom's listless address to the group. "Don't get me wrong, I'm totally grateful for my angel's safe arrival. But I so badly wanted a natural delivery," she confessed. "I can't shake my disappointment over the C-section. It's not what I wanted for either of us."

The facilitator stood at the front of the room in tranquil

command, rhythmically patting the perfectly packaged bum of the babe in her arms. She must be Ellen, who had emailed to introduce herself last week.

"I understand, Lindy," she responded with the kindest of eyes. "Thanks for sharing, and we'll be talking about how we reflect on our babies' births."

I rolled my eyes and hoped no one saw. I knew I'd needed to get out of the house and interact with people other than Matty, but Kumbaya group therapy wasn't what I was looking for. The scene could easily have been mistaken for an AA meeting or grievance support group had it not been for the presence of the brand-new humans, cozy blankets, and binkies. Back to the baby in Ellen's arms, she hardly looked real with her coordinated couture ensemble and pink headband. Tights on an infant whose diaper needs to be changed with relentless regularity? While the majority of the ladies' faces around the table were drawn and desperate—reflective of only a couple hours' sleep—one mom stood and swayed outside the U, looking like the next appointment on her calendar was a modeling shoot. You wouldn't have fathomed that she had recently grown and given birth to a full-term, bouncing baby boy, but the evidence was in her arms.

Finally stepping into the room, I felt myself blush and was relieved to spot an open seat quickly. I got settled without attracting too much attention. Ellen welcomed me as she continued the discussion. Fidgeting a bit—at least Matty wasn't hollering like he did the one other time we'd been in public—I unfastened him and lifted him over my shoulder in case he needed to pass gas from one end or the other.

I wasn't the only late arrival. Someone else rolled in just behind me, but she had an excuse. She had two brand-new humans to corral. Seemingly without embarrassment about her tardiness, she parked the double stroller in the back corner, skillfully removed both carriers, and gracefully squeezed all three of them between two other women and their little ones. She was far more confident than I, and she had double duty. Pun intended. I thought to myself that if presented with the opportunity, I'd ask her for her secret. Which books had *she* read? The stack on my bedside table was about to topple, and my brain didn't have room for one more parenting theory. Even so, I obviously missed something because we were a mess.

I sat there fully prepared to not fit in and plotted my early exit. After about 15 minutes, however, I tuned into what was being said. Kind of like a kaleidoscope coming into focus, I listened. Most of the other moms were also breastfeeding, and a couple talked about their worry in not knowing exactly how much milk their baby was getting at each feeding. I had the same concern. One gal was eager to begin sleep training before her pediatrician recommended it. So was I. And my ears really perked up when Cate hinted at her resentment toward her husband's business travel.

The irony in the class's name, "Transitions to Motherhood," wasn't lost on me. There was no transition at all to my new, strange life; it was baptism by fire. I mourned the normal life I had just weeks, days earlier. Processing the room's chatter, my body softened into the chair. I no longer had one foot turned toward the door. I didn't share anything myself, yet on some less-than-conscious level, I sensed that I was exactly where I needed to be. Maybe the group would transform my total trepidation of motherhood into some semblance of peace, even confidence, in this new role. I told myself not to get too excited or too hopeful.

As the session came to an end, I came back to reality and felt like I was back in high school. I didn't know if I should stick around and make small talk or bolt home. Matty was a ticking timebomb and would need to eat soon. I made eye contact and smiled at a few of the ladies then quietly made my exit. In the lobby, I ruffled through the diaper bag and all my pockets, but the valet ticket was nowhere to be found. I checked again and again. The wetness returned under my arms, and heat flooded my entire body.

"Hey there," someone said, coming up beside us with her stroller. *Great timing. I'm feeling really social right now.*

"Oh, hi," I said. "Where did you park? I used the valet and can't find the ticket. Seriously, I'm a disaster."

"I actually found street parking around the corner. Couldn't believe it," she said. "Here, why don't you leave the little guy with me and go talk to the people at the desk? You're not the first person to lose your ticket. What's your baby's name again? My memory is worthless these days."

"Thank you so much. He's Matty, Mateo, and I'm Brie. Will you remind me of yours?" I asked.

"I'm Sarah, and this is Ryan," she said. "Go, go, and we'll be right here waiting."

The security officer and desk staff were nicer than nice, as if their sole purpose was helping moms who lost their parking tickets. I was suspicious of pity again, but maybe it wasn't really the biggest deal. Maybe I needed to get used to being the person who loses things.

"All set?" Sarah asked as I hurried back.

"Yep, thanks again," I said. "I feel like such a loser. This having a baby thing has kind of knocked me hard, if I'm honest."

"Me, too," she laughed. "I guess you wouldn't know it, but I don't usually leave the house in my slippers. It took all of me to get here, and I totally forgot my shoes . . . and my purse."

"Ha! I wouldn't have noticed if you didn't say anything. Thanks again for your help!"

"Yeah, of course! Will you be here next week?" she asked.

"Yep, see you then." *I guess I was coming back.*

In those 75 minutes (90 minute class minus my tardiness), I felt less alone, I heard my story in other women, and I met someone I could see myself potentially being friends with.

The ride home wasn't as quiet as the ride in. Matty unleashed, making his case for food as soon as we hit the road. I tried to focus on the lake, its azure color reflected by the sun and clouds. I couldn't hear the music over the bleating screams. I knew I was pushing it by not feeding him at the hospital, but I couldn't risk the subsequent diaper change and spit up in public. Matty and I paid the price for the next 20 minutes, but at least we wouldn't have witnesses to the madness.

The three flights of stairs were an extra workout with leaking breasts and a wailing baby. Nearly immune to the screams, I powered through to change his diaper before feeding him in the hopes that he would fall asleep eating...and stay asleep. Matty nursed on both sides, a delicious reward for both of us. In the second miracle of the day, he let me put him in the crib. I was rarely able to put him down without a protest, and I was too tired to contemplate what I'd done differently. What I did know was that the sleep experts wouldn't approve of nursing Matty to sleep. At that moment, I didn't care. Truly didn't care.

One of the ladies had shared her secret of letting go of the untidy house and sleeping when her baby slept, so I gave in. I didn't trust the monitors, so I dozed off in the nursery glider. It felt like a bed at the Four Seasons. Nick, the cat, jumped into my lap, and in that moment, all was well. We'd done it! We went into the world, a step toward a return to normalcy. Matty was okay, and I was okay.

* * *

I'll always remember that scary, stressful, and ultimately successful outing as a glorious glimmer of hope. That day saved me because it made me realize—it made me FEEL—that I wasn't alone in the craziness of what had become my life. I consider myself to have been a married single mom. I'll unpack that a little. Javi and I dated for four years and knew we wanted to have kids soon after getting married. The plan was to try on our honeymoon. That was, until everyone kept telling me it could take a while after having been on the pill for 15 years. Well, it didn't. I was three months pregnant at our April wedding and spent the occasion stone-cold sober amongst our less than sober friends, none of whom were married, let alone expecting. I should have seen the lonely road that awaited me.

I was happy. I wanted nothing more than to be a mother, so the absence of umbrella drinks on our honeymoon didn't bother me. I loved every minute of the anticipation and read a book a week on pregnancy and how best to prepare the house and myself for our new arrival. I read about breastfeeding, when to introduce a bottle so Javi could participate in feeding, all the types of bottles and nipples, feeding schedules, sleep schedules, infant "playtime," developmental stages, and on and on. I had a personal library of books, and I shopped avidly according to authors' recommendations. You might say I was a little impressionable, the perfect consumer. I shopped for clothing, organic bedding, brain-stimulating toys, strollers, and gadgets that generations of women before me survived without.

I convinced Javi to join me one Saturday to complete our registry, but other than that, I was shopping solo or with my mother. From the very beginning of our marriage, Javi worked 24/7, building a new business. I quickly learned not to take his absence personally, but it hurt a little more when he didn't even make time for our growing baby. When he did come home at a decent hour, I tried to engage him in what

I'd learned and purchased. Alas, not even a martini could inspire his convincing interest in the matter at hand. Each and every decision about how we were going to parent was mine.

Everything was ready by late September, and I was two weeks overdue. My doctor was watching me closely and wasn't going to let me go much longer. I warned Javi to keep his phone close ahead of an ultrasound appointment. Sure enough, I had virtually no amniotic fluid left, and I was sent straight to the hospital for induction. I called Javi with the news that we were having a baby that day and that he needed to go home and get my bag before meeting me at the hospital. As he wrapped up calls and rescheduled meetings, I checked myself into Labor & Delivery. Every other lady sitting in a registration cubby had a partner. I was used to rolling solo, but that instance of solitude felt like one of those huge theater spotlights shining directly on me for the world to see. Swollen fingers had forced me to remove my wedding band weeks earlier. Feeling acutely and deeply alone, I wondered what people thought.

I'd endured an hour of a Pitocin IV and increasing discomfort when Javi waltzed into the room and immediately caught the nurses' attention—even the male one—with his charming words and gestures. Everyone liked Javi. I liked Javi. I just wanted more of him in our life together. We were blessed with a smooth delivery and experienced only one concerning complication. Matty aspirated meconium (early stool he had passed in utero, likely attributable to being past-due), which required immediate attention and treatment to avoid severe illness. Both Javi and I remained calm and handled the situation well. In the end, and with the knowledge and gratitude that Matty was perfectly healthy, I was relieved that Matty had been the one to move his bowels during delivery, not me. Truth be told, pooping on the bed was one of my biggest fears going into childbirth. There were enough indignities involved without that.

My first hours with my thick, dark-haired boy were the best of my life. I felt joy in a way I'd never experienced. I'd loved Matty since I learned I was pregnant and had been exacting in my care of the two of us for 42 whole weeks. It's hard to find words to describe the joy; it was intense, vast, and unadulterated. I expect one element of it was utter relief in having a healthy baby with 10 fingers, 10 toes, and a good APGAR score. I will never take that miracle for granted.

More practically, the timing of my induction and the ensuing eight-hour labor caused me to have lost the entire night of sleep. The next day passed quickly with visitors and so many opportunities to practice nursing and diaper changes. Javi is the youngest of his parents' three sons, and his brothers were way too excited to carry on the tradition of taking the new father out for a few drinks. The operative word being "few." They showed up early in the evening after the grandparents had departed. They pretended to be interested in meeting Matty and congratulating me but swiftly whisked Javi off to the local establishments. I wasn't overly disappointed initially, as the peace of just Matty and me in the room and the call button service of the nurses felt luxurious. But at Javi's disruptive return, my emotions raged. I had strongly encouraged him to take a cab home and sleep there. But always one for optics and impressions, he was going to stay that first night at the hospital with his wife and new son.

The loveseat in the room barely accommodated his smelly, drunk, snoring self. Painfully tired myself but unable to enjoy a substance-induced sleep because someone needed to tend to the crying baby, I hoisted myself out of bed with the guardrails. Walking to the bathroom was a chore thanks to a cramping belly, pulsating crotch, and the horribly uncomfortable disposable underwear and massive maxi pad that somehow missed most of my hemorrhages. Still, I refused to push the call button and run the risk of someone observing the dysfunction in my early hours of motherhood. If someone else saw it, I might have to admit it. Clearly, I was in this alone.

We were discharged the next day, likely only because no one entered the room before Javi was showered up and fresh as a daisy... the doting dad. I felt like an invalid being pushed to the car in a wheelchair, and it hit me hard that no license, no specific credential *at all*, is needed to become a parent. I was terrified and didn't see how Javi and I would be successful in sustaining our small creature's well-being. Since infant car seats are installed in a rear-facing position, we couldn't even see Matty crying as we drove home. We had gone from being one entity to two, and not being able to see him felt counterintuitive, even though it was the safest way for him to travel. I'd entered Mama Bear mode, and everything was a concern. Everything was worrisome.

The condo was exactly as I had left it when I headed to my final ultrasound appointment. My half-full coffee cup was still on the counter, and a highlighted, dog-eared copy of *What to Expect When You're Expecting* was on the island. Like a history museum exhibit, the scene confirmed how life was just two days prior. As soon as Javi placed Matty's carrier on the table, Nick (the cat) jumped right on up. His tail immediately puffed, and the hair on his back stood up straight. I'd never seen that reaction from him, being an indoor city cat without many natural stimuli. I'll never know whether Nick's instinctive reaction was rooted in his feeling threatened, defensive, or excited. Whichever it was, I could have said I was feeling the same. Further, I believe Nick knew on some level that life would be forever different from that moment on.

Javi went back to work as soon as I got settled at home with Matty. Back then, people went to the office, and working remotely wasn't really a thing. I was left to figure everything out on my own. I've always held mixed feelings toward Javi's career. It's easy to carry resentment around his choices of prioritization and his domestic absence, but his success and the fact that I could stay home with our children were two things I was really happy about in our marriage. I didn't want to work professionally and didn't care about not applying my graduate level degrees. My new job was taking care of Matty, and I've always been grateful that I could do that full-time. In time, Javi's work felt more like a conflict of interest than an act of love to provide for our family. It became a big wedge in our marriage.

It's not until you embark upon something meant to be a shared partnership experience, like having a baby, that some of us realize the partnership is not really there at all. Matty was the quintessential example of something Javi and I created together. In such a union and mutual responsibility, you're meant to rely on the other person. But I couldn't rely on Javi as my co-parent.

For me, the isolation of motherhood was a slow burn. As a result of none of our other friends being married or yet parents, it began even ahead of Matty's birth. Going out to the bars got more and more awkward and ultimately unenjoyable. The wine bars felt slightly more appropriate, but places like McGee's and Barley Corn's and all our Wrigleyville haunts were no longer where I belonged. When I stopped showing my face on the weekends, Javi stayed home with me a couple times. Eventually, I told him to go out because there wasn't any sense in his missing out on the fun just because I was. I didn't have to say it twice. I preferred to be alone in the evening anyway; it was what I was used to. Occasionally, friends would stop by on their way out. I always served them a drink or two, but those visits became briefer and less frequent. What we had in common was dwindling, which made me sad.

My early weeks with Matty are a blur; sleep deprivation has an amnesic effect. Most everything I did was in reaction to something Matty did. I craved order, consistency, a schedule, and the ability to plan anything at all: a coffee or lunch date, even a phone call. Once Matty was six weeks old, I got serious about implementing Dr. Marc Weissbluth's theory. As a pediatrician and renowned sleep researcher, he authored what became my bible, *Healthy Sleep Habits, Happy Baby*. I've always been a pro at following instructions, so I figured his step-by-step guide to a good night's sleep was my return ticket to sanity. I fastidiously followed his every instruction, from early bedtimes and tactics to help Matty self-soothe to rigid consistency around nap times and coordination of feedings with sleep and awake time. I logged Matty's every sleep, including how long he cried and how long he was quiet.

The theory was highly prescriptive and got excellent reviews. So why was it so difficult for me? Each time (which was nearly every time) the evening didn't go according to plan, I was shattered. I know that sounds dramatic, but that's how I felt. Like a failure time and time again. First it was about me not doing it right. Then I felt myself getting mad at Matty for not complying and behaving as expected. Sleep training made my life even smaller, and the walls felt as if they were closing in on me. I wouldn't leave the house at nap time, which could really be any time according to the signs Matty was supposed to be giving me. Dr. Weissbluth preached that sleep begets sleep, so I had to be available for Matty to nap in his bed (not in the car seat carrier or stroller) whenever he was ready. So, I spent my entire days watching him and assessing his readiness to sleep based on eye rubs and fussiness not attributable to hunger or a dirty diaper. No day was the same, and the collected data did not lead to predictability as promised. We both cried a lot.

One day I found the courage to meet my best friend Heidi for lunch in an opportunistic window of 90 minutes when Matty was supposed to be awake according to our schedule. We stayed local so we could walk and avoid the hassle of city parking. I must have looked at my watch every 10 minutes for the entire lunch. I'd packed a bottle of expressed breast milk, hoping Heidi would be willing to feed Matty so I could eat a proper meal. I was also following the instruction of spacing feedings with sleep so Matty wouldn't develop a dependency on feeding in order to fall asleep. This seemed like one of the more important tenets of the good doctor's theory. My fixation on the time was also tied to getting Matty home without his falling asleep in the stroller. Sleep in motion (in an electronic swing, car, stroller, or being walked or swayed in my arms) was not considered "real" sleep. This is why I couldn't enjoy lunch or my stroll home on a beautiful fall day in magnificent Chicago. I was constantly striving for better and constantly concerned about what was going wrong. Was he eating enough? Sleeping enough? What did each cry mean? Which was the hunger cry? Which was the tired cry? Was he pooping enough? Too much? My head exploded with questions and guidance, and much of the information I took in was contradictory. I was left feeling confused and like my nerves were exposed to the air. It was painful; I was in pain.

Javi knew nothing of my state because he wasn't often around to witness it, nor did he ask. In his defense, I wasn't talking about it either. A casual observer wouldn't have pegged us as unhappy or disconnected. We showed well. I didn't recognize at the time the part I played in the distance between us. All I knew was that I had nobody. Javi managed to check most of the husbandly boxes and would arrange for his mom or my mom to come watch Matty so we could sneak out to dinner. Every few weeks he'd have flowers delivered. I would have preferred 30/70 on diaper duty, or a shoulder to cry on (or punch) as I let Matty cry it out at bedtime. But I did appreciate the gesture of flowers, even if it was shamelessly tied to the goal of reconvened intimacy. At one of our dinners out, he alluded to as much, which piqued a new concern in my mind. Sex had not even come close to crossing my mind. I didn't crave it physically or emotionally.

Javi's reference to his desire was not only a surprise, but it also felt like an insult. Nonetheless, as soon as we got home and I'd checked on Matty, I went straight to the bathroom.

I can't believe I did this, and it's even harder to believe that I'm sharing it. I used a hand mirror to look at my genitalia. The postpartum bleeding had subsided, and I was no longer using pads, an enormous freedom. But that did not mean I was hot to trot. I was entirely unprepared for what I saw. My vaginal opening was still as wide as a quarter. I was shocked and horrified to see that things were still flapping in the wind. The visual was what I needed, however, to remind myself that I wasn't ready. I wasn't ready physically and was even less ready emotionally. Javi could take care of himself in the shower. It was fine by me.

I don't recall the event or when it eventually happened. I must have blocked it out. Sex felt like another responsibility, an obligation to Javi, not something I wanted for myself or at all. We were losing, or had already lost, the emotional intimacy of a genuine connection. I didn't have a drive or need for physical intimacy. I was depleted. I was taking care of Javi, in addition to Matty, the house, the dog, the cat, the laundry, and everything else. But who was taking care of me?

My new support group at the hospital ended up taking care of me. The ladies were like an outsourced parenting partner, diminishing the loneliness in my marriage and in my early motherhood. I was hooked after the second meeting. I knew that I wouldn't be besties with every one of the women, and that wasn't the goal. The instant and mutual respect we developed and held for each other was a great gift, and I'll always believe that that group saved me. It allowed me an awakening around what it meant for me to be a mother. I was no longer alone. Each week one or two of us would break down, and I don't mean light tears. I mean sobs demonstrative of deep emotion spanning the spectrum from elation to despair. I was saved by honesty, vulnerability, camaraderie, and the physical respite provided by a couple of volunteers who were there for the sole purpose of holding our babies to give us mommies a little space to talk.

Between meetings and at the conclusion of the formal class, we gathered a few times as a full group, meeting at one of our homes or a park. I could call any one of those women at any point, high or low, and I didn't have to worry about being judged. I knew that whatever question or concern I had would be received and considered with compassion. Naturally, smaller groups within the full group began to form. I connected most quickly and easily with Sarah. With the exception of my being a stay-at-home mother and her working, we had a lot in common. We planned evening strolls with the boys, and eventually, Javi and Doug got to know each other so the six of us would get together for a weekend cocktail. I wasn't looking to swap out any of my long-time friends, but Sarah and I were on the same page, living a similar track of life. As it happened, we've been close friends ever since and went on to share the experiences of three children each. Our budding friendship was a life-saving connection that helped me start to win.

One of my biggest wins was the evening I fed Matty at 5:30 pm, got him in jammies, read a story, and put him in his crib awake. He fussed, no real crying, for about 15 minutes and eventually went to sleep. On his own! No rocking, no nursing, no holding the pacifier in his mouth so it wouldn't fall out. He did it. I did it. We did it. Sex might not have been memorable, but Matty soothing himself to sleep sure was! I cleaned up the kitchen, put in a load of laundry, and sat down on the couch with a glass of wine. At that moment, I felt successful on behalf of both of us. I felt hopeful. I felt like an adult again. The big picture hadn't changed. Being a married single mother still felt like the weight of the world at times, but sleep helped!

All my efforts were for Matty. He hadn't asked to be here;

he was our creation, and I would do anything for him. Looking back, I realize that my work resulted in a reward greater than I could have ever imagined. Perhaps my pride is a little grander and my chin a little higher because I did it myself. I don't know what I missed not having a collaborative co-parent, but it all worked out because while I did it myself, I wasn't by myself. I had my tribe.

• • •

My advice for new mothers feels a bit cliché, but I mean it from every piece of my heart and soul. Know, if for no reason other than my telling you, that this time will pass . . . the beautiful and the uncomfortable. It will all pass. So, breathe in your baby's sweet scent. Linger in the moment with him because everything else that needs to happen will eventually get done. Don't feel guilty about holding your baby so he sleeps. It's okay! Maybe you both need it. Cuddle so close that you can inhale his warm exhale. He won't ever be this small again, not even tomorrow. Caress his head with your lips. Hair or no hair, it's a guaranteed rush. Look deep into his eyes, really deep, and tell him you love him and that you both will be alright (even if you don't yet believe it). Don't stress too much about any one thing, milestone, or challenge because I promise it will eventually be a phase in the rearview mirror. Before long, you'll be on to the next thing that has you worried and obsessed.

Please try to trust that your baby, your daily life, and your relationships are evolving as they should. Admit the hard and confront the difficult. Hold onto the soft and see the wonderful. As the adage goes, the days are long (sometimes very long), and the years are short. History dictates that you and your baby will eventually sleep in "normal" patterns. And believe it or not, one day, you'll panic because your child is still napping after three hours.

In time, he'll have a girlfriend or a boyfriend and prioritize them. But today, beautiful today, you are his entire world. It's weighty, and it's also a tremendous honor. If you're feeling sad, scared, confused, mad, or lonely, call a friend. Preferably one who has had a baby, but anyone will do. Just call. Get out. Go for a walk or to the coffee shop. Your baby's fusses don't bother others the way you worry that they will. Unless you're at a fine dining restaurant, which you likely are not. Find and attend a new mother's support group. There are ladies there whom you need in your life.

I researched and studied more about motherhood than for any other test I've ever taken. Yet, I felt the least prepared that I have ever been. And this wasn't a test! It wasn't a dress rehearsal. It was the real thing, with real consequences, from Day One. There was no room for a learning curve. I endured, I persevered, and I survived. I could have more than survived in the early days if I hadn't been so alone. You don't need to be alone. Please don't be alone.

As an important closing note, I don't wish to vilify Javi. We've addressed our marriage over the years, and he continues to believe we approached it correctly. He stands by our agreement to tend to our respective parenting "lanes," managing the household and working for a living. I will give him that we did make such a pact, but I suppose I didn't realize that the lanes would be so rigid and so deep. The lanes became trenches with very little common ground in between. He trusted me in my roles, and I trusted him in his. Perhaps that's why he didn't feel the need to help at home. At the time of this writing, we're in the midst of a divorce. It's amicable and reasonable. Sure, grudges exist, but they don't add up to general regret. Together, yet separately, we created, supported, and raised three remarkable young people. For that, I love him and always will respect and appreciate him as well. Now, it's time for me to put myself closer to the top of the priorities list. From this vantage point, I know I can effectively do that at the same time I continue to enjoy and support Matty, Marley, and Willa on their respective journeys. There is enough time and room for all of us.

Chapter 8

Doctor's Orders

MEREDITH

"A season of loneliness and isolation is when the caterpillar gets its wings. Remember that next time you feel alone."

—Mandy Hale

Introduced by mutual friends our senior year at University of Michigan, Pete and I were young Wolverines in love. I fell quickly for his gregarious spirit. His smile spanned his face, from his pearly whites to his sparkling eyes; the smile was infectious, a spell. It was impossible not to feel at ease, embraced, and entertained in Pete's presence. We were a harmony of opposites: a charismatic business student from Chicagoland and a taciturn pre-med student from rural Michigan. It worked. We worked. Our focused dedication to our respective fields required flexibility, patience, and cooperation in growing and maintaining our relationship. We supported and loved each other through the trenches of undergraduate study and eventually post-grad work and all of life's happenings. We had a propensity for making careful, considerate, and effective decisions. The decisions about when to wed and when to have our first child were no exceptions.

We planned our wedding at the conclusion of my pediatric residency. Logistics were complicated, including work, the all-too-early passing of Pete's mother, and the hospitalization of his father the week before the wedding. Even so, we relished the event itself, our honeymoon, and the start of our official life together. From early on, our busy calendars meant that time together—date nights, weekend meetups with friends, and jaunts to the lake—required advanced scheduling. Pete's dad lived on a mid-sized lake in Northeast Wisconsin, and we stole away there every chance we could for a dose of the water's serenity, the scent of pine and wildflowers, and reduced distractions. Toward the end of our second married summer, baby discussions boomed. We were both feeling the itch, but we needed to sort through careers and other priorities before committing. I was the newest partner in my then small-ish, male-dominant practice and was very focused on not compromising my contribution to the team. Pete was leading a start-up venture and was confident in his ability to balance his high-energy work with fatherhood.

One summer evening, we watched from the dock, toes dangling in the water, as the sun dipped low on the horizon. A canvas of reflected trees mirrored in the calm water.

"Mere, let's do this." Pete leaned into my shoulder. "I can't wait any longer to start our family."

"Yeah, everything seems to be in order," I said, my eyes set on a sailboat in the distance. "I think I'm ready too." I couldn't analyze my readiness more than I already had, and suddenly, it felt so definitive. We were no longer speaking in hypotheticals. I was ready. I responded to his lean with a longing look up into his eyes.

"It's a plan then," he said, pulling me in for a long hug.

I felt myself flush. "By this time next year, there will be three of us!"

"Oh, no." He pulled away and looked at me funny.

"I'm confused. You just said you're ready."

"I know, I know. I am. It's just—let's think about the timing a little more. Let's get in one more summer at the lake. You know, lazy dock days and boat rides. One more summer."

We had our plan, and we were blessed to get pregnant quickly. My partners at work were supportive, especially when I promised to work until I went into labor and to return after only eight weeks. I'd walk from my office, which was on the hospital campus, to Labor & Delivery and call Pete on the way. I'd be one of those moms who grows and delivers a beautiful baby and whose upgraded life as a mother proceeds without much disruption. I saw it all the time with my patients.

Only my pregnancy with our daughter, Sophie, didn't quite work out that way and instead was stressful from nearly the get-go. At 17 weeks I began experiencing contractions. My OB had the challenge of championing the safety of my pregnancy in the context of my drive to maintain a rigorous work schedule. I took medicine, attended frequent office visits, and complied with a modified work plan. I did everything I was told to do out of grave fear of delivering a pre-term baby. That would not be me. No way, no how. I could not have survived that guilt.

A few weeks later, the conversation got even more real.

"I'm sorry Meredith. We can't do this anymore," Dr. West said. "You need to get off your feet entirely."

"Got it. I promise to sit longer between patients, and I'll see if I can cut my hours back a little more, so my days are even shorter," I said.

"I don't think you're hearing me," she said. "I'm saying that you can't work anymore, not at all. Modified bedrest. I'm sorry."

"I can't. I can't stop seeing patients now; they need me," I appealed. "I can't walk out on my partners either. I need to work. What else can we try? A different med?"

"Meredith," she said sternly. "I'm calling it. You need to stay home and keep this baby inside you. Doing anything else puts you at risk of premature labor that we may not be able to stop."

That was all I needed to hear. My patients needed me, but in my new reality, so did my baby. My baby needed me to stop, so I stopped. But by God was it hard. I became the patient, and the role reversal was jarring. I didn't sit around well on a good day, after having worked 10 hours and gone to yoga class. The days at home and off my feet, growing and protecting my girl, were reallllly long. One can only read and watch daytime TV for so long. I was a doer, and there wasn't much to be accomplished from the couch and bed. My parents and sister didn't live locally, and everyone else I knew was at work. I dreaded Pete leaving for the office. I talked to my belly, but the renter in there didn't talk back. I talked to myself more than seemed healthy, and worse, from time to time, I caught myself talking to someone who wasn't actually there. I came to understand how imaginary friends might be conjured up and to appreciate how they would be better than no friends at all.

The Summer Olympics in Sydney saved me. I had always loved gymnastics, but that summer, I mastered the rules and regs of archery, pentathlon, and handball. I also became well-versed in the Australian lifestyle and all the swimmers, of course. The United States brought home 37 gold, 24 silver and 32 bronze for a total of 93 medals that year, and I like to think my fandom from the couch had something to do with it. Each dose of the drug I took to curb the contractions had an effect similar to that of an espresso or two. So, my cheering was impassioned. When Olympic coverage paused for a newsbreak, my mind crept right back to the tangle of guilt in abandoning my patients and partners. I longed for the day that I could care for *everyone* again. I allowed myself to begin a countdown at 37 weeks. Each evening, I valiantly crossed off another day survived.

When I went into productive labor at 38 weeks following

multiple false alarms, my body did its job well and delivered to us Sophie Marie, named after Pete's mother, Ann Marie. My gratitude for Sophie's health and safety and the wonder of brand-new life coursed through my every cell. I saw and touched babies every day at work, but this was entirely different. The precious one in my arms was mine. Her silky head, trusting eyes, and rosy, plump lips set hooks in my heart. I would always protect her. Her fingers wrapped around mine felt like an earnest thank-you for every boring, maddening, anxiety-ridden moment on the couch and in the bed. Those torturous weeks at home were behind me, and our next beautiful chapter was upon us.

I spent the first several days post-delivery pacing the house to quiet Sophie. After being sequestered to a sedentary existence for so long, I vowed never to take walking for granted again. Pete returned to the office quickly. Loneliness pecked at me, but I wouldn't let it in. I had Sophie; I wasn't alone. I was living what I had waited so long and so hard for. Only she was a tough baby. My milk supply wasn't great; I fed her, and she continued to cry. I figured I'd nurse, and it'd be easy, that I'd be successful. I wasn't expecting this really fussy, though adorable, baby. My vast clinical knowledge, training, and years supporting patients' families didn't convert to even a consideration that my own experience would be so nerve-wracking.

I look forward to doing for my daughter what my mother did for me that November when Sophie was two weeks old. She was a grandmother-in-residence for a week, my companion in pushing through the difficult feedings, enduring the grating crying, and holding Sophie so I could get some sleep. Of all her acts of mothering and grand-mothering, that week goes down as the most heartfelt, roll-up-your-sleeves, and unconditional love my mother has provided me. Upon her departure, I cried in symphony with Sophie.

We had moved to the suburbs based on the requirement that

I live within 15 miles of the hospital associated with my practice. My friends were still in the city and didn't yet have children, and I didn't know the families in our cul-de-sac well. I was back to being by myself all day, Monday through Friday, 7 am to 6 pm, back to solitary confinement. I was well educated on babies, how they work, and what's normal. I knew that while Sophie was fussy, she was healthy. It was me who wasn't thriving. Folded laundry and blankets piled up in the bassinet and crib because Sophie didn't inhabit them. She slept only when held. So, that's what I did. I held her all day long. As soon as Pete walked in, he was handed a fussy baby, often damp from my sweaty chest. At least he had the commute from the office as transition time between a hairy workday and an unsettled homestead. Two hours of Pete and his help weren't enough, but I took it. In addition, a couple bouts of mastitis required me to be the patient again, calling my doctor for antibiotics.

"Other than the breast infection, how's everything going?" Dr. West asked. "Is Sophie a good baby?"

"Oh, yeah," I said. "She's a champ. Things are going great." I made note of the falseness of my report.

One complication of being a pediatrician-mom was my desperate need for Sophie not to get sick. What would my partners think? To control against that disaster, I limited her exposure for two full months. Perhaps "limited" is a little soft. I didn't take her anywhere and let very few people into our home. If an infant under two months of age develops a fever, it means an ER visit and possible admission to the hospital. I'd been through that with patients, and the guilt of Sophie potentially getting sick as a result of my seeing a friend or going to lunch was too great. We spent Thanksgiving alone, and despite the tempting magic of showing off a Christmas baby, we stayed home for Christmas, too. Pete's father was sick, and my nephew had chickenpox. Quick no. It was acutely disappointing and sad, but the holiday wasn't without gifts. Pete and I made a surf and turf dinner on Christmas Eve, and by someone's good grace, Sophie slept in her bassinet and didn't cry until after the Yule Log. A Christmas miracle!

By January, I was ready to return to work. I felt guilty that I didn't find joy in my days at home being a mother. Where was the intense bonding? I looked for the joy, but it wasn't there. I was stuck at home, alone all day with a fussy baby. I craved a routine . . . and the opportunity to hand a crying baby back to its rightful owner and move on to my next assignment. We had planned on sending Miss Sophie to one of the highly reputable local daycare centers. It's easy to believe that given my line of work, I should have known to put my name on a list when I learned I was pregnant. But I didn't, and there were no openings. I was petrified as we interviewed nannies. It was such an intimate thing to have someone in our home—our nest—taking care of *our* baby. It felt risky, exposed. Would she invite her friends over? Look through the cabinets? The closets? What if she got frustrated with Sophie when she cried? My father, who has always offered the very best advice, encouraged me by saying, "There are good people out there. Don't always anticipate the worst." Dad's commentary allowed me to open up to finding us the perfect partner in caring for Sophie.

I knew I needed a very calm, grandmotherly figure, since Sophie was so tough. Jane fit the bill: early-60's, grey hair, and straight from England, the archetypal British nanny. A couple of weeks later, Jane confessed that she expected ours to be a cushy job, with only one child and a nice couple.

"Now I understand why there's a TV in the nursery," she said. "This baby only sleeps if you're rocking her! Not sure what I'd do without the soap operas." The TV's placement was one of Pete's more brilliant ideas.

Jane's feedback that Sophie was a feisty one validated that

it wasn't just me. My days at the office allowed me the break I needed and provoked my joy in taking her into my arms at the end of the day. The joy *was* there. The joy showed up when I got myself back, and that happened when I returned to the office. I jumped right into being the pediatrician I knew. I returned in a full-time capacity because I've never been a half-way kind of person. The return to the identity I knew had me flying high until its clash with my new identity couldn't be ignored. I was no longer solely a pediatrician. I was a pediatrician-mom, and that second title wasn't a sub-title. I wouldn't let it be the second fiddle job, the side gig.

I tried my darnedest to figure out how to pump and still be one of the guys. It was important to me that my new circumstances didn't draw unnecessary attention. Most peds practices keep long hours in order to serve—and spend adequate time with—all our sick and well patients. My time was tight; in fact, there was no time between patients. I attempted to pump at lunch, but the dairy collection didn't go well. There were conflicts everywhere in my efforts to be so much to so many. My worlds collided, my priorities were torn, and my body didn't know what to do with all of it. Pumping at my desk, under a tremendous time constraint, didn't exactly send serene messages to my milk factory. I nursed Sophie when I was home, but it was never enough. I would supplement after nursing, and she got formula from Jane during the day. I did the best I could.

I had been out on bedrest and then out on maternity leave and was making up for lost time. The last thing I was going to ask for was *more* time to pump. I immediately fell back into my hyper-efficiency persona, ensuring that every patient was cared for before taking time to get Sophie her food. No one did anything wrong, but I had no professional role model, no one to demonstrate how I could feed my baby AND work. I was just doing my job and didn't see how low on the totem pole I had placed myself and my new baby. After patients, after my partners, after medical record notes, after everyone and everything. And mine wasn't just any workplace—it was a pediatrics practice for goodness' sake. Three years later another female partner who had come up through the ranks had a baby and advocated for herself. Boy, did I admire her. Today, every woman (physician, nurse, administrator, everyone) who is breastfeeding gets extra time in her schedule to pump. We've come a long way.

Sophie was about four months old, and I had given up nursing altogether when Pete convinced me that he needed me back. I had just gotten myself back, and now *he* needed me.

"Come on, Mere," he persuaded. "We need a break. I miss you. Let's run away just for the weekend."

"I don't know," I said. "Jane isn't available on the weekends."

"You know your parents would flip at the chance to come stay with Sophie."

"Mom doesn't know how we do things, and I just feel like something's going to happen while we're gone." I knew my pushback was futile. When Pete gets fixated on something, he almost always gets what he wants.

"I need you too, you know," he said, the way I imagined a puppy dog might speak. "You're my wife, not just my buddy in paying the mortgage and calming a crying baby."

He had a point, but his words didn't move me.

"She'll be absolutely fine. But if something does happen, we'll be able to get home quickly." Not the most reassuring answer.

I played along the best I could. In the end, Pete sold me on a trip to Orlando based on the direct, 2.5-hour flight, and I agreed so as to not to hurt his feelings. What did hurt was my stomach. I realized at the gate what a blatant error we had made. Mickey Mouse ears everywhere, toddlers wiping their noses on anything they could find, and parents strung out before vacation even began. Orlando, really? What were we thinking?

As soon as I could fire up my laptop in the hotel room, I was booking a return ticket for the next day.

"What the heck, Meredith," Pete said as he peeked over my shoulder.

"I don't care what you think," I yelled, a rare occurrence. "I'm a mother, and I need to be with Sophie."

"And *I* need *you*," he said, similarly inflamed. "It's been a long time, a really long time, since we've been together, alone."

"Pete." My voice cracked, and I began to weep. A new guilt swept over me.

Nothing can compete with the biological and psychological drive to be with and take care of our children. Separation is painful and proved to be way worse than I even imagined it would be. Child rearing is so time-consuming and emotionally complicated, and then our partners need us and want us back, and there's guilt around that. We only have so much capacity. But that wasn't a conversation I could have had with Pete at that moment. Instead, I dug deep, said a few prayers, and bought tickets for Epcot, the most adult venue available at Disney. It's the only good memory I have of that trip, feasting our way around the world. Amply distracted from the pain of separation, I was able to have fun with my husband, temporarily.

Our weekdays were chock-full. My expanding practice demanded a full-time-plus schedule, as did Pete's entrepreneurial venture. Jane was the third leg on the stool of love we crafted for Sophie. We became a well-oiled team, in constant communication coordinating comings and goings, food on the table, and as much consistency as possible. Each of us flexed where we could, and we always held Sophie as our central emphasis. When she was about 18 months old, Pete and I managed to stop long enough to get pregnant again. From the day the ultrasound revealed we were having twin boys, my heart ballooned at a rate akin to their cells' rampant proliferation. The world was tinted blue. The anticipation of double joy elated us. Jane seemed to take the news as well as could be expected; her job was soon to get much less cushy. I worried about whether she'd hang around. But she loved Sophie, and we were generous with bonuses, so I remained hopeful.

I didn't let myself obsess over a potential reoccurrence of preterm contractions. Even so, double trouble reared its head at 13 weeks this time, bringing our team to a screeching halt. Concern was higher with a multiple pregnancy—everything times two. Two lives were at stake, and the associated guilt of risking their safety was twice as paralyzing. The medical management of the situation was more intricate. We played around with several pharmaceuticals, but I experienced low blood pressure, causing me to feel dizzy and generally "off." My unsteadiness wasn't safe for any of us, so we opted against the meds. My doctor's orders were for strict bedrest for the three remaining months of my pregnancy, a bad dream. I rose only to use the bathroom and then was right back to lying flat. With my spending 24/7 there, the bed wasn't the delicious haven it used to be. It was a soft, warm prison. No couch, no summer Olympics. Three months of winter's darkness in bed. I didn't feel well; it was hard to concentrate on reading, so I watched a lot of TV.

Sophie was with Jane during the day, and they went on adventurous, educational excursions. But when they were home, Sophie wanted to be with me. We watched Disney movie after Disney movie. Ariel, Pocahontas, and Jasmine will always mean something a little bit different, a little bit more to me than to most. Sophie learned the power of her voice quickly, as she yelled downstairs for Jane to bring snacks. There were no exceptions to my quarantine. If Pete had to work late and Jane couldn't stay, we had to line up additional help in the evening. My helplessness and inability to independently care for my daughter were not only saddening but also maddening and frightening. I watched from the window as life went on without me. I developed insight into the lives of those with chronic diseases. The malaise was constant. The drastic limitations and singlehanded onus of protecting the twins felt heavy.

The only occasion on which I was permitted to leave the bed, other than to use the bathroom, was a doctor's appointment. Getting dressed was a big deal and no small victory. The boys and I had grown quite large because I was such a rule follower (still am). Truth: I was gigantic toward the end. Maternity clothes didn't come in our size, and I wore the equivalent of a weightlifter's belt to hoist my belly up where it belonged. We were a sight! The brief time spent vertically felt wrong and had me on pins and needles. Kind of like being at the dentist and waiting to feel the drill, each step I took had me anticipating contractions—contractions that *I* would have caused, that would have been *my* fault.

Upon being sent to bed the second time, I promised myself that if I managed to keep the twins inside me until they were fully baked, I would enjoy them once they were out, no matter what. That meant that I wouldn't let crying or sleep deprivation get to me. I envisioned the beauty of nursing them together. To avoid the typical complications of twins, Dr. West decided to induce me at 37 weeks. As with Sophie, my body executed the birthing part of the project very well. I delivered the boys naturally after four hours of labor. Weighing 7 pounds 9 ounces and 6 pounds 6 ounces, respectively, Leonard William's and Maxwell Edmund's arrival was the most liberating event of my life. I was instantly lighter, literally and figuratively.

Despite the chaos, I was in a much better place mentally with Leo and Max than with Sophie. I channeled my inner Olympian and hooked a baby up to each breast, which was more of a bicep and forearm workout than I was fit for. I propped them with pillows and contorted my body to support their latching, but it felt like a choking hazard in the end. If one baby fell off a nipple, the other needed to burp by the time I got him relatched. I gave up that dream and pivoted to nursing one baby and bottle-feeding the other in the bouncy seat. That felt like a choking hazard, too! Eventually, I succumbed to feeding one at a time, and it was loud. Babies' cries are in a high-frequency range, which is the scientific reason for their startling effect on adults. Leo was always fed first because his screams were more piercing. I'd nurse him on one side, put him down, then nurse Max on the other side. But it was never enough, so I had to bottle-feed both of them anyway. The stress of the never-ending cycle and Sophie's synchronous meltdowns affected my letdown. It's really no wonder I never had enough milk, but I didn't give up. It was important to me that the boys received breastmilk for at least as long as Sophie did, so I again pumped when I could upon returning to work.

I called Pete with strict instructions as I was leaving the office one evening. "Don't feed them until I get home," I instructed. "I have the goods!"

"Meredith, these boys are starving," he said, voice raised over their wails. "Really, you want me to wait?"

"Yes, I'll be there in five minutes," I huffed.

I hustled in and handed Pete the treasure bag. "Just this?" he looked past me to my briefcase for more inventory.

"Yep, it was busy today," I said in explanation, almost nonchalantly. "This is all I got."

"It's two ounces. Do we split it, and everyone gets an ounce?"

My reaction could have gone either way: defensive or mutually humored. Luckily, that day, I was able to laugh. We both did.

"Yep, give 'em each an ounce of mama's brew and then formula," I said.

Pete and I were better with expectations the second time around. We knew we were outnumbered, and we accepted the crazy. It was still overwhelming, but our nervous systems had been through it before.

"Let's assume we'll get nothing done," Pete suggested. "And if something does get done, then it's a good day, a bonus."

Although a great departure for me, it was a stance we needed to adopt to survive. It allowed us levity and grace most of the time. Pete tried so hard to support me and all three kids, but he wasn't so successful by night. I'd breastfeed one twin and counted on him to bottle-feed the other. One night I had just nursed Leo, and I went to check on Max and Pete. Out cold in the rocker, Pete was indeed "feeding" him. The only problem was that the nipple was in Max's ear. Max was such a patient baby and rarely cried, even with a nipple in his ear. Pete got off easy on that one.

Going from zero to one child was hands-down a harder transition than going from one to three. The math doesn't make sense, but my first postpartum stint was one of the most alone, most isolating times of my life. Life as I knew it came to a sudden stop. It shook me to my core and took me by complete surprise, and no one prepared me for the loneliness and the grief I felt for my former existence. I do wonder why we aren't prepared for this change. Why isn't it talked about?

I've been asked how being a mother has made me a different doctor and how being a doctor has informed how I mother. While these questions feel big, the answers are pretty straightforward. I don't believe I changed fundamentally as a pediatrician upon becoming a mother. I hope I've always been compassionate and never overly dogmatic. Most of the new mommy tears I see are around matters of breastfeeding or the endless efforts to keep a fussy baby calm. Although I always promote breastfeeding as the best nutrition, there are times when mothers aren't able to fully breastfeed. If supplementing with formula is necessary for any of various reasons, enjoy the closeness of nursing and the distinct high of feeding your baby from your bountiful body, and then top her off for some additional nutrients until she's comfortably full. How beautiful an opportunity. And if you tried breastfeeding and it didn't work, then you indeed tried. Sometimes our bodies don't cooperate. Similarly, while I do recommend that parents try not to hold their babies *all* day long, some babies need more holding to be calmed. But moms do need breaks, and getting your little one to nap in a bassinet or crib is usually better for everyone and a much-needed breather.

While I may not have changed clinically as a pediatrician, I will say that my firsthand experience as a mother was likely a factor in my more proactively opening the important conversations. I've always felt for new moms coming in. I see how worn out they are. In addition to the exhaustion, I see distress in their wanting everything to go swimmingly. There's too much pressure for everything to be perfect. This has been the case for centuries, and the ideal has become even more pronounced, no doubt due to social media and other opportunities to put forth perfection. There's immense pressure to look perfect and to say it's perfect. Anything else feels like failure. I've never had a mother say that she's not enjoying her baby, and I've been doing this work for more than 25 years. I know moms are feeling and thinking different things, but making that statement to a doctor feels risky. I didn't even say it to my own doctor when I was the patient. Please know that we want you to share, we want to listen, and we've gotten better at facilitating the conversation.

Routine pediatric visits are brief; 15 minutes isn't enough time to cover what's going on with Baby *and* how Mom is faring. Our profession as a whole has gotten better at asking mothers, "How are you doing emotionally?" We now screen for Postpartum

Depression for the first six months via a tool called the Edinburgh Postnatal Depression Scale. We should have been doing this a long time ago, and I'm so glad we're doing it now.

As for how being a doctor influenced how I show up as a mother, I was not immune to the standard struggles. I'd say mostly it's humbled me and honed my gratitude for my own children's health. My heart goes to the mothers of children with significant medical problems, and there have been many days when I embraced my babies tighter than I might have if I were in a different profession. There have also been moments when knowing too much (clinically) hindered my trust in believing that I know what's best for my children simply because I'm their mother. I've never been cavalier in my double title of pediatrician-mom. I've consulted Pete and reached out to my partners regularly over the years. I encourage all new mothers, regardless of their education or profession, to reach out to partners, friends, or colleagues for input and perspective.

From the rearview mirror, I regret having returned to work full-time after both pregnancies. I can make myself feel better and justify it by thinking about the patients I helped and the little lives I impacted on those long days away from my own little children. Pete and I probably could have made my working part-time possible, at least for a period of time. At the same time I have regrets, I'm gentle on myself because it's who I was in my life at the time. I did the best I could.

Fortunately, I was relinquished from my active guilt when I dared to ask my kids as young adults about my work when they were younger. Their responses were quick and consistent: they have fond memories of family evenings and weekends. We planned carefully around my call schedule and always made the most of our time together, enjoying nature and local attractions whenever possible. They also remember enjoying school, having fun with Jane and friends after school, and participating in dance, sports, and Boy Scouts. They didn't cite feeling slighted. Rather, they specifically commented on their recognition of the importance of my work and how much I loved it. Needing more, I pressed further, and they reported not to have ever felt that my love for my work trumped my love for them. They claimed to have always felt valued and prioritized. They granted me retrospective permission to have done life—and motherhood—my way. Sophie must not have been too scarred because she is soon to begin medical school herself. The boys appear to be following in Pete's footsteps, pursuing careers in business and technology.

In conclusion, I'll leave you with a few gentle suggestions that I share with my patients. Think of them as "Doctor's Orders."

- Figure out what works best for you. Let go of comparing your situation to those of others. You know best how to care for *your* baby. Trust your instincts, do the best you can, and partner with your pediatrician, as necessary, to bolster your confidence in your baby's wellness.

- Expect that it's not going to be perfect, and that's okay. Even if something isn't perfect, it can still be very right.

- Call your OB if you're not feeling right—physically, mentally, emotionally. It's okay to admit that you're struggling. Don't be afraid to say your experience isn't good, that you're not in a good place. There is no shame in it not being easy, and you are not alone!

- Ask for help. We all need breaks. Heartening help and remarkable resources are available, but sometimes you need to ask. Make a list of friends, family, and neighbors. They will most likely be overjoyed to lend a hand.

- Call your pediatrician even with the seemingly silliest circumstances. If it gives you peace of mind, we want you to call! We want you to come in.

- Join any variety of new mom groups. Hospitals, churches, and community centers often host or know about such forums. Whether in-person or virtual, it's always cathartic to hear, "Yes, the same thing happened to me."

Chapter 9

The Gift of Signs

NICOLE

*"Faith and fear both demand you
believe in something you cannot see. You choose."*
—Bob Proctor

It was almost fun at first. A super consequential scrapbooking project or big deal résumé requiring a perfectly finessed portrait of qualifications. Todd and I carefully crafted our profile book to captivate expectant parents and influence their choice of *us* as the parents for their baby. We documented our education, living arrangements, and religious beliefs. But how could we describe in words the love we would have for an adopted child? We felt as confident as we could about our self-promoting portfolio. That was until six months went by with no interest. Did we choose the wrong photos? Was my career intimidating? Had I taken the wrong angle with the "Dear Birth Mother" letter? Were we too casual in our attempt to be approachable?

I knew I was meant to be a mother, as many women do. But justifying on paper that I was the best on the market was an exercise I don't wish upon anyone. Competition was high, with

30+ families vying to adopt any one available child. We had grown accustomed (but not numb) to the continuous passes, to the ongoing rejection. Even so, the voice persisted in my Monday morning meditation. "Adopt, adopt, adopt," it said. Always seeking the guidance of signs, I put that one in the bank.

Campus was humming with returning students and faculty. The light snow and residual sparkle of the holidays fed the collective energy. I've always loved the head of a new year: a new beginning, new promise, and new hope. I loved floating between classrooms, checking in on my faculty and students. As the director of the Nursing program at a major university, I was constantly on the move. Glancing at my phone, I found three voice messages, a rarity. One from my dentist's office with a second reminder that I was overdue for a cleaning, one selling me a new automobile warranty, and one from the adoption agency. Thanks to transcription technology, I didn't actually listen to the first two and jumped straight to the third.

Hi Nicole. It's Deborah. I hope your Christmas was lovely and Happy New Year to you, Todd, and your fur babies. Call me as soon as you can please. I want to send your book out, but I'd like your consent first. There are some nuances involved. Anyway, give me a call.

With only seven minutes left before my next meeting and a hefty walk to the conference room, I called Todd.

"Hi, Hon. Do you have a second? Are you sitting down?" I asked, speaking as fast as my feet were shuffling. "Deborah wants to send our book to someone, a young Native American woman. She wanted to confirm with us before sending it."

"Great news, but why'd she ask?" he replied. "We told her we're open to any nationality, didn't we?"

"Yes," I said. "But do you remember the deal with tribal laws and how we'll be on the hook for even more money? I'm not concerned, but I still wanted to check with you before calling her back." The Indian Child Welfare Act is a federal law that protects Native American children's connection to their indigenous heritage and culture. Full of intricacies, it requires non-Native American adoptive parents to meet strict eligibility requirements and jump through lots of hoops, often involving attorneys and their fees.

"Absolutely yes, tell her to send the book," he said. "We'll figure out the finances. But Nicole, please don't get your hopes up, Babe."

"Believe me: I can't, and I won't," I said. "Gotta run to a meeting. Love you."

I passed our permission to proceed along to Deborah and finished my afternoon meetings. Fighting the enigma that is Cincinnati rush hour traffic, I counseled myself the way I would a friend, reminding myself to balance my own heart's protection with the faith that if I kept it open, another heart would find mine. Even if hope felt too tangible or too risky, I could draw on faith that things would work out.

Deborah sent everything to the birth mother the next day for overnight delivery, so Wednesday could have been a day of anxiety, knowing we were being examined under the magnifying glass. Fortunately, the day's busyness at school distracted me from focusing too much on what would predictably become another "no." Todd and I went out with friends that evening; we had gotten pretty good at distracting ourselves.

By Thursday, I had all but put the scenario out of my mind. My phone rang as I approached the gym to burn off some steam.

"Hi Nicole," Deborah said. "It sounds like you're driving. Are you able to pull over for a second?"

"I'm pulling into a parking spot now," I said.

"Great, because I have amazing news."

"No, I don't believe you."

"Really, Nicole. The birth mother, Stacy, picked you guys," she said.

"Oh my God, oh my God," I exclaimed. "No way. Okay, I'm going to call..."

"There's more. She's in labor and on her way to the hospital."

"Oh my God, oh my God," I repeated. "We don't have anything ready—no nursery, no supplies, no baby clothes. We thought we'd get to meet the birth mother and would have time to prepare. What am I supposed to do?"

"For now, not a lot," she said. "Go talk to Todd, try to stay calm, and I'll provide updates as I receive them. Assuming all goes as planned, we'll start the paperwork soon."

How was I going to do nothing while my future child was being born a few states away? "Got it, thanks. I know this baby is coming into this world. Still, I can't get my hopes up that he or she will be ours. Right?"

"One step at a time," Deborah said. "She chose you. Let's focus on that and keep breathing. I'll be in touch."

I took to saying the Serenity Prayer on a continuous loop, at times audibly, other times in my head. Todd and I made dinner and watched a show, and as we made the laughable attempt to sleep, we received word that our baby girl had arrived safely. "Our baby girl" had such a special ring to it and was an answer to so many prayers. Although I'm not at liberty to divulge the details because of privacy clauses within tribal adoption policies, we had reason to believe that Stacy might change her mind.

We had to rise above our frantic concerns and proceed anyway. It was a good thing I didn't have to be on campus Friday because I was intermittently paralyzed. We went back and forth with the agency a few times, not knowing the phone calls and pulls on our hearts were only the base of the administrative and emotional mountain ahead. I retrieved the shopping list from the folder Deborah handed us the first time we met her. To shop for diapers, onesies, bottles, and burp cloths was to open ourselves to receiving a baby, which was, in turn, opening ourselves to heartbreak. I couldn't, and I didn't, shop that day. Instead, I cleaned. I controlled what I could.

I imagine that everyone going through the adoption process holds the fear of the birth mother changing her mind. It seemed insane to put ourselves through the stress of the unknown with Stacy, but what choice did we have? We'd wanted children and weren't able to conceive naturally for years. This baby was here, and she was relevant and dear to everyone involved. I didn't know if I was strong enough to face the situations I'd seen working as a nurse in the NICU: these babies both brought families together and tore them apart. Even if Stacy did change her mind, I would have to be happy for her. A baby was born! My utterly conflated heart didn't know how to feel, how to proceed through the emotional quagmire. So, I put one foot in front of the other and responded to the next steps as they were doled out.

While we were able to put off shopping, we weren't able to stall on naming this child by the next morning when we would start the paperwork. Our friends were already planning to come for dinner, so we toasted with them and eventually set out to determine a name. We hadn't received any photos, and it was challenging to think about a label as personal as a name without having a visual. I Googled photos of Native American newborns as inspiration. Not exactly a fair assessment, but it was the best I could do. We laughed at ourselves and tried to celebrate that nothing about our journey was conventional.

"When did you decide to adopt anyway?" Shea inquired. "I never asked your plans because I didn't want to pry. I just figured you guys weren't going to have kids."

"Ah, it went like this," I sighed. "As the years rolled by and we weren't getting pregnant, I had no desire to pursue fertility treatments. I didn't want my body to be a lab, and I didn't want to become a prisoner to the schedule. Adoption was on my heart from very early on."

"Me, not so much," Todd shared. "It was foreign to me. I didn't know anyone who'd adopted."

"Obviously, he came around," I smiled. "We could have spent our baby budget on fertility, and we all know there's no guarantee there. Or, we could spend the same amount of money on adoption and be more likely to get a baby." Instead of chasing fertility treatments, we chose to spend the money on a life that was already in process. We were fortunate to be able to pursue this path to parenthood.

"Todd, what changed your mind?" Shea asked.

"Not entirely sure," he admitted. "I guess once we moved into this house it felt like something, or someone, was missing. So, we proceeded with the home study. I think eventually the idea of a baby in need got into my head. It became clear to me that we could help. And that he or she would, in turn, help us."

"So, what are we going to do about a name, people?" I asked, looking at my watch. We needed a name in the next 12 hours.

Over a couple of hours and some bubbly, every name I liked was a quick "no" for Todd, and vice versa. Eventually and, upon tensions rising, Todd threw out, "What about Aria?"

"What does the name mean?" was always my first response. Todd pointed at the search results on his phone.

"The Hebrew meaning is lioness of God. It also means air and has a melodic quality to it," he explained.

"Done, I love it," I said. "I can't believe it."

"Amazing," Todd said. "You pick the middle name."

"Easy. Grace," I said. "Aria Grace, may you be ours, sweet girl."

Saturday had us signing the initial paperwork and making the upfront payment, which was more than even the adjusted financial expectations. With the price tag a moving target and without a cinematic suitcase full of money, we had to get creative in securing the next installment. And we couldn't procrastinate on shopping any longer. We descended upon Babies R Us. The filling of five shopping carts began systematically and evolved to our slap-happy (alright, maniacal) selves tearing up the list and grabbing whatever seemed like a necessity. In 90 minutes, we had the staples! Thanks to credit, we'd have some time to figure out how to pay for the large load. My friends had all been thrown multiple showers and spent weeks carefully building their registries based on product reviews and word-of-mouth recommendations of sanity-saving supplies. Obviously, there was no time for such ceremony in our circumstances. With our new possessions in hand, we went on to prepare ourselves for the inter-state drive the next morning.

I came down from the day's whirlwind, the first time I had stood still in hours. We were told to plan on living in Aria's birth state (which, again, I'm not at liberty to specify) for at least a month. It would possibly be more, but we knew it would be at least that long in a hotel room with a newborn, due to Native American and other adoption laws. All the typical considerations came to mind: it would be colder there; I wouldn't have in-room laundry; we'd need to eat all our meals out. But then snuck to mind the reason *why* I was packing; it was not your typical road trip. *What if we drive all the way there and it doesn't work out? How will I take care of her so far away from home? What if we fall in love with her and have to leave her?*

As I spiraled, a deep sense came over me, a sense that God doesn't bring you something He's not going to get you through. My intuition roared that I wouldn't be alone. I had a vision of people around me. Another sign? It was much more than a premonition, and the idea of being supported was pertinent because Todd would have to fly home each week for work. In a way similar to the morning meditation voice I'd heard telling me to adopt, I received a very timely message that things would work out. When my parents came over that evening with baby-related offerings and to lend their support, my mother must have sensed my need to hear that message of faith in human form.

"Honey, I know you're worried, but you're going to be great. I know it happened fast, but you guys can do this," she said and wrapped her arms around me for a long, tight hug.

We said our goodbyes and didn't sleep a wink for the third night in a row. By 2 am, I succumbed to insomnia and got up to clean the oven and microwave. A couple hours later, I fell onto the couch and dozed off briefly. I cuddled the only babies I knew, the dogs. I told them what little I knew about Aria and promised not to abandon them.

Not even a week after receiving *the* call, we hit the road for the one-and-a-half-day trek. I would have driven one and a half weeks, one and a half months, any length of time and highway to meet my baby. We spent Sunday night in Small Town, USA. Monday morning, we drove the final stretch and stopped by the hotel to set everything up. Jo, the hotel's marketing manager, checked us in and knew why we were there. I read the kindness in her eyes, a stabilizing force amidst the chaos.

Todd and I played house, only we were at the Extended Stay Suites. Not a huge fan of hotels, I was pleasantly relieved by the newer construction building and generously sized sleeping, living, and kitchen spaces. No funny odors or strong air fresheners; everything seemed clean. We scurried to set up the Pack-n-Play featuring a bassinet and built-in changing table. Todd literally pulled at my shirt, eager to get to the hospital, but I wanted to organize the diaper station and wash the bottles and nipples, so we were ready for anything when the three of us returned as a family.

I pinched myself as we arrived at the hospital. This. Was. Happening. The operation wasn't as organized as it could have been, but I wasn't there for five-star service. I was there to claim my baby. The social worker assigned to us, Sally, was cursory in her explanation of what was about to happen. She promptly swept us from the reception desk to the room where Stacy was waiting for us.

Sitting in an armchair at the window, she glowed. Our eyes locked immediately. I wouldn't say she smiled, but her mouth did move. Her eyes were swollen but dry, stoic. She rose as I approached tentatively, and I reached out my trembling hand to grip hers. Against the suggested protocol and without thinking, I hugged her instead. My rehearsed words failed me, so I embraced her with intense love, profound admiration, and abundant appreciation. It wasn't exactly like hugging a steel pole, but her reciprocal squeeze wasn't quite as impassioned. Logic told me she had chosen me as the mother of her child, yet I craved even the smallest indication that she liked me.

She asked us a couple questions that weren't covered in our profile book, and I handed her a gift and a letter I'd prepared. I was desperate to interpret her emotions, but I wasn't getting any hits. I wanted her to like me enough to give me her child, but I also didn't want to seem like I was trying too hard or to do or say anything that would make her change her mind. That scene remains my very best example of having zero control over one of the biggest opportunities of my life. I continued with the Serenity Prayer. As the conversation lulled, Sally asked if the three of us would like our photo taken. Stacy agreed, posed, and then made an announcement.

"I want to go see her again," she said and walked to the door.

My insides dropped just as painfully as if I'd been on an actual roller coaster. Sally hopped-to and followed Stacy out of the room without addressing us. We were her clients too, but we were left alone in the small room to ruminate. Todd paced like a caged animal, mumbled to himself, and occasionally blurted a rhetorical question.

"What does that mean?" he asked. "Why does she want to see her? This can't be good."

I spoke calmly. "Todd, she met us and now probably just wants to go see her. Maybe she wants to say good-bye. I think it'd be weird if she didn't."

"Well, this wasn't in the plans, and I can't sit here and wait for this to unravel," he said. "Didn't she sign the paperwork? If we came all this way . . ."

"The agency did tell us that she's allowed as much time as she wants," I said. "They need to be sure that she's making the right decision for herself. Better for her to take the time to come to that conclusion now than to get a call two days from now, at least that's the way I see it."

Just as we were about to open the door to find her, Sally returned. "Stacy's going to spend some time. When she's finished, you'll be invited to the nursery to meet Aria. You can stay here, or you can leave, and we'll call you."

Insufficiently distracted by our phones and each other, we left to drive aimlessly around the town we didn't know. I focused on the fact that Sally was still speaking as if we would meet Aria, as if she would be ours. But Todd couldn't get there. He felt the unbearable weight of waiting to hear that we were (still) going to become parents that day. His fury heightened to the point of calling the agency against my suggestion. I didn't want his tirade to result in the agency changing its mind about us. Their hands were tied, however, and there was nothing they could do. Deborah's counterpart talked Todd down and was at least able to confirm that this does happen in many cases. As a bonus, the heated exchange helped kill about 15 minutes. What in reality was only about an hour total felt like an eternity until Sally called us.

"It's time to come meet your baby," she said.

"Tell us exactly what's going on," I said. "I don't think we can take any more surprises."

"Stacy signed the paperwork and is on her way home," she explained. "Get on back here!"

"Okay, we'll be right there. So, we'll be able to see Aria now?" I confirmed.

"Yes, it's time," she said. I reached for Todd's hand, and we drove in silence.

We met Aria in the hallway because she'd already been moved from the nursery. I peeked over the plastic bassinet as if squinting at a fine figurine in a museum display case. Just to be sure, I checked the card on the end. Aria—9 pounds 7 ounces. It was her! Our daughter. I was a mother. Well aware of the rules and protocol, I asked permission to hold my baby. I pressed her cheek against mine, inhaled deeply, and held her against my racing heart. In that moment, we became one. Despite her not having grown in my uterus, I was hers, and she was mine. Careful not to invade the moment, the nurse shepherded us into a private room where Todd reminded me of his presence. Seeing Todd hold her melted me. He was a daddy. Continuing my investigations, I lifted the thin pink beanie to see if she had hair. If she had hair! I was immediately envious of her thick, lush locks. I would learn the ins and outs of styling her hair, which is so different from my very fine blond hair.

The high of meeting her was fleeting, as my mind reverted to scanning for what to worry about next. We were on top of our paperwork and payments. Stacy had signed her paperwork, therefore commencing the 72-hour window in which she could change her mind. My chest felt heavy. *Was this going to turn out to be a glorified babysitting stint? Maybe this isn't what God wanted after all.* The Serenity Prayer no longer did the trick, and I turned to breathwork to center myself. We had made it that far, but I still felt so vulnerable.

Todd and I were eager to get on with things, as if leaving the hospital's confines would somehow protect and cement our new titles and responsibilities. However, the nurse had a checklist to fulfill: demonstrate that we could feed her, show that we could change a diaper, and place her in a safe sleeping position. At some point, Todd could no longer bite his tongue and assertively assured the nurse that I knew very well how to do all these things, suggesting we get a fast pass out of there. To no avail.

I've been asked if I felt prepared for motherhood, especially given my profession (in addition to all the classes only adoptive parents are required to attend). Yes, I was prepared to care for her physically. But from a life-change perspective, the answer is a big NO. I was not prepared. I don't think anyone is ever prepared, especially when it happens in five days' time.

I unwrapped the hospital-issued blanket as we finally packed up and were about to put Aria in the just-out-of-the-box car seat carrier. At the seam, amongst the pastel bears, read CINCINNATI in small black print. The signs kept coming: Aria was meant to be with us in Cincinnati. Years later, I learned that those blankets are manufactured in Cincinnati. At the time, I was just grateful for another sign.

Aria belonged with us; it was exactly the reassurance I needed to carry on. I made every effort not to let the incessant fear of having her taken out of our arms and hearts get in the way of our first days together. I didn't want my guards against potential devastation to interfere with our bonding.

* * *

Todd visited on the weekends, earning my endearing reference to him as a helicopter dad. He has always taken his role very seriously, and Aria had him pegged from the very beginning. Competing demands prohibited extended family and friends from traveling to visit us. Perhaps if we had been at a Marriott Vacation Club beach resort, we'd have seen them. In seriousness, Mom was tending to my grandmother, who was ill. Understandably, she felt guilty leaving her mother. I've wondered, however, whether Mom keeping her distance may have been her own way of eluding the fear of attachment, just in case anything unraveled. We all fell hard for the promise of Aria.

So, it was Aria and me, just the two of us, figuring out our new life together. She had lived in utero for nine months in one energy and was thrust into an entirely new energy (mine) in a transient living space. I had lived almost 40 years focused primarily on myself, with dedicated fragments of my attention allocated to Todd, family, friends, and work. I was pretty set in my ways: I ate at this time; I watched this show each night at this time; I went to bed at this time; I worked from this time to that time; and I went to wine night with the ladies on this night. Life quickly fell into two buckets: before Aria (BA) and after Aria (AA).

I can't say that meeting her basic needs was very different or harder than I expected. She was an easy baby, and I somehow always felt resilient. She ate well, and the fact that she drank from bottle nipples and not my breasts wasn't an issue for me. I delivered sustenance to her, she enjoyed it, and I was joyous. She was a good sleeper, waking at a reasonable cadence to do reasonable things like eat and be snuggled back to sleep. Middle-of-the-night crying spells did perhaps grate on the nerves more than they would have had we been at home. I worried that she might wake the neighbors. If she did, I never heard about it. Reruns of *Golden Girls* on the Hallmark channel got us through.

I'd say we were pretty darn patient with each other and our respective learning curves. I kept an open mind when it was clear that she hated being swaddled despite the literature and every other baby I'd met. From the first week, her preference was to stretch out and have her bare tootsies exposed. And Aria went with the flow, enduring baths in the undersized sink and the rigmarole of the laundry room. We got very efficient at packing up the stroller and timing wash/dry cycles around eating and sleeping. She was also patient with me, a new mother and fish out of water. Through the good days and the hard days, we did photo shoots in new outfits and sent the pics to everyone back home. We weren't alone. Our community of fellow hotel dwellers felt like a warm blanket. Each of us had unique reasons for our residency there, yet we were cohesive, and I believe we were meant to be together in that place at that time.

One advantage of not having given birth and not breastfeeding was that I could indulge in wine at daily Happy Hour in the hotel lobby. When we made it down, Aria was passed around, everyone loving on her. The vision I'd had of people being around me proved to be not only accurate but divine, indeed. One of the families was transferring to the area from Texas. Erin and her three-year-old daughter, Ella, were at the hotel during the day while her husband, Gabe, was at work. Erin's and my budding relationship was orchestrated way in advance; I just know it because it turns out Ella was adopted. Erin was generous in sharing details of their process, helping me see that others had survived our same rollercoaster ride.

Despite my disconnection from my normal life, I reflect now on our month in the hotel as a beautiful bubble of bonding, between me and Aria and between acquaintances who became angels. Jo, the marketing manager who had checked us in, arranged my first appointment of many with the notary at the local bank and accompanied us to take care of Aria while I completed the piles of paperwork. If I didn't make it to breakfast, she would have a plate sent to the room or bring it herself. Between her and Erin, I had someone to watch Aria so I could shower. Erin commiserated with our regular visits from the social worker. We were being carefully watched and scrutinized, and I didn't want to make a single mistake. I wanted to be sure I was doing everything right: completing paperwork, checking more legal boxes, paying the next installment, trips to the pediatrician, etc. More quickly than I expected those weeks to pass, it was time to leave our initial nest and head to our real home.

I didn't take the maternity leave offered to me, which sounds crazy when I say it now. While the Deans did find coverage for a couple of my classes, I figured that staying engaged and participating in Zoom calls would anchor me and provide some sense of normalcy. That proved to be true during my month away with Aria, but stuff got real upon returning home. It was more than typical re-entry pain following an extended vacation. I was cast into the deep waters of taking care of Aria, establishing her permanent nursery, taking care of the dogs, accommodating everyone's desire to visit on a whim, and keeping up with professional responsibilities. I probably should have gone back to my superiors at that point and taken the leave. But my people-pleasing ways had me striving to be everything to everyone; I knew no other way. I see now that part of me figured I hadn't given birth and so didn't really deserve the break. In my previous jobs in Labor & Delivery and the NICU, I'd seen medically complicated births, and I'd seen very sick babies. That wasn't us, so I could keep doing everything I had always done and simply layer on the tasks associated with caring for a baby.

People commented on just how good I had it, mostly working from home with my newborn but out of the house two or three days a week with a built-in babysitter in my mother. The one thing Stacy made us promise was that we would never put Aria in daycare. If anyone watched her, it would always be family. We have honored that to this day. Yes, I was fortunate. But anyone who has done the juggling act knows that the one whose care goes unattended is your own. It may look manageable on paper, but in reality, it isn't sustainable.

When Aria was only three months old, I had to take a business trip to DC. I was torn. How could I choose my work over my baby? Did I even have a choice? Not really, if I wanted to keep my job. My mother encouraged me to focus on how my presentation would benefit all those in the audience. My mother has always been very convincing, and she would be there to cover for Todd as necessary. It was a Sunday morning departure, which anyone who travels for work knows is awful. I cried saying goodbye and the entire way to the airport. I nearly turned around at every juncture: getting on the toll road, parking at the airport, and checking my luggage. Money was so tight due to having overextended ourselves with the adoption that I checked the balance on the credit card to be sure I'd have money to grab coffee or lunch. The university pre-paid the hotel stay, but incidentals would fall to me until my expense report was paid.

There wasn't a seat assignment available for me when I checked in, so I was told to approach the agent at the gate. My historical experiences with gate agents had never been positive, but that morning, Laurel engaged me with a smile. She assigned me a seat, handed me my updated documents, and wished me a good flight. I reclaimed my spot against the wall with the goal of being close to the front of my boarding group. I'm typically Group 4 or higher, but my boarding pass read Group 1. How odd, I thought, realizing my seat was close to the front of the plane. Maybe it was a regional plane since it was such a quick flight to DC, or maybe there was a bulkhead or emergency row seat available at the last minute.

I walked aboard and was confused to find that Laurel had put me in First Class. I had never flown First Class before. I guess she knew I needed a nap to recharge and mend my breaking heart after walking out on Aria. I received a beamed message from above: it was time to take care of myself and pamper myself, and my First-Class seat assignment was my sign. In that moment, I sat up straighter and set out to make that trip special. I cannot explain the shift. It just happened. Normally, I would have sat in my hotel room and refined my presentation, giving my entire evening to my employer. Instead, I walked around exploring our nation's great capital and expanding my personal horizons. I treated myself: I put myself first, and I slept. I felt full in a way I hadn't since I'd become a mother.

But my return home was a return to the hamster wheel of caring for everyone but myself. It took a year and a herniated disc in my neck to force me to stop saying "yes." I was stuck in bed for days with no choice but to let others help. Those days of humble self-reflection resulted in my vowing that my life would look much different going forward. I'm grateful for that damaged disc as the catalyst to my stepping out of roles that no longer served me. Motherhood altered my priorities, and I transitioned away from the pulls of academia to start my own coaching business.

I believe we are all sent messages from the Universe and that it's our job to be open to hearing them. We must listen. We must watch. To receive a sign is a divine point of guidance relieving us from carrying the weight of the world, figuring things out ourselves, and making all the decisions. The signs I was blessed enough to receive around Aria allowed me to repeatedly choose faith over fear and to subsequently and truly know that how life was unfolding was exactly as it should.

The signs that appeared to me may not be the same signs that appear to you, and these were mine:

- That voice to "Adopt, Adopt, Adopt" provided me with faith that I would become a mother in exactly the right way for me, Todd, and our baby.
- The vision that there would be people around provided me with faith that I wouldn't be alone in my early days as a mother, so far away from home.

- The imprint of Cincinnati on the hospital blanket gave me faith that we would survive the 72-hour waiting period and that Aria would be ours.

- My seat assignment gave me faith that I would find a way to adequately care for myself, as I cared for Aria and tended to my various other responsibilities.

* * *

To anyone who might believe that adopting is akin to special ordering a baby and commanding the situation, the notion couldn't be further from the truth. Our path to permanent custody of Aria was long and winding and, at times, stormy and petrifying. Following months of actively waiting for a birth mother to choose us, she was born to us in January. Following those tortuous initial 72 hours, fearing that Stacy would change her mind, we began our beautiful life together and eventually rooted at home. Still, the technicalities continued, including Stacy's required legal surrender of Aria twice in each of two different states under different state laws (so that the tribe could never come back and take her from us), multiple attorneys in multiple states (cha-ching, cha-ching) and the appointment of Aria's own child advocacy attorney. Finally, her adoption was finalized in Buffalo, NY, in November.

All that said, the stresses, the headaches, and the blatant lack of control were all very much worth it. We believe Aria came to us very intentionally and despite the legal and procedural complications, our connection with Stacy has always felt like a loving one. While Aria's adoption was closed (as opposed to open), we have had some connection with Stacy. I've always let my intuition guide me around what I share with her. I know her heart and curiosity desire to see and know that all is well with Aria. As a mom, I share what I feel another mom would want to know.

She made a life-changing decision, and I will always honor that. To this day Aria loves staying at hotels. She gets super excited and loves the smell. I think she remembers.

I will never take the privilege of motherhood for granted, and I am exceptionally grateful to share the title of "Mom" with you. Please be sure to take care of yourself amongst all the other people and things you tend to. We are better for others when we are strong ourselves. Lastly, please remember to place faith over fear, and when that's hard to do, look and listen for the signs.

Chapter 10

Close Call

CORA

> "Stop trying to control life.
> It gets in the way of divine intervention."
> —Cheryl Richardson

This feels like a massive confession. To whom, I'm not sure. Perhaps to my son, maybe myself, possibly God, potentially my husband, and likely all of the above. A confession and an apology. For what, I'm not quite sure. For being selfish, irresponsible, short-sighted, flippant, and/or egotistical? Again, likely all of the above. My hands are trembling as I begin to write. This is scary, but here it goes. I'm sharing at the risk of judgment, and with the great hope of connection and catharsis.

Life was good that summer. Sam and I were fulfilled by our jobs, our home and community, and our two happy, healthy boys. Mac and Carter were four and a half and three years old, and there was nothing left to want. We had just stamped the decision that we were finished having children. A thoughtful conversation and audit that spanned several days confirmed for us that we were extremely blessed. We decided to stop while we were ahead. While we didn't know what we were missing not having a daughter, we weren't going to create a new life for the sole purpose of trying for a girl. Girl or boy, we didn't see how another child could uplevel what we already had. We were happy, very happy.

The following week was vacation. We returned to one of our favorite cabin resorts a couple hours south, where the days were always more laid back and relaxed. Very little can beat a sunny, mid-70s day on the lake, the kind of day Sam refers to as a "chamber of commerce day." The air, the water, the trees, and the dragonflies have a way of clearing the concerns and pressures of everyday life. Basically, it's utopia. And in that spirit, I spontaneously re-opened the kid conversation on the boat one afternoon.

Are we really sure? Maybe I could see one more bambino on the boat. I think we have enough love for one more. Should we keep this vibe going and add one more to the party?

Sam humored my follow-up chatter, but in the end, we held onto logic and reached the same conclusion. Our family of four was whole. No reason to be selfish when what we had was perfect. I've always preferred even numbers anyway. Fast forward to naptime the next day, and I apologize if this is too much information. I wasn't interested in returning to oral contraceptives after Carter was born. I didn't want the hormones, so the plan was that Sam would have a vasectomy once we had made the final decision that we were finished. Part of his incentive to schedule the "Big V" was the cumbersome use of condoms, especially at our age. It was on his long to-do list.

The boys were asleep, and we were sun-kissed, carefree, and clad in skimpy swimwear ... lake life. The opportunity presented itself, and we took it. We were always efficient; our time windows were often brief due to the boys. As we heated up, Sam told me to hold on while he went to grab "coverage." I told him not to, to just pull out. Neither of us was a big risk-taker. After confirming with me twice, we proceeded, and he did pull out. It felt rebellious but not illegal. I immediately proceeded to the bathroom to wipe thoroughly, however, just for extra measure. I didn't dwell on it or really even think about it afterward. Following five days of bliss at the cabin we returned home, where real life resumed and reoccupied my mind.

A couple weeks later I started feeling crampy, which was typical for me ahead of my cycle. Some months I had cramps and other months I didn't, but I was always like clockwork: every 28 or 29 days. So, by 6 pm on Day 28, I became slightly concerned. I recalled that with my first pregnancy I had cramping that early and had mistaken it for menstrual cramps, to the point that I popped a couple Advil, poured a glass of wine, and took a bath. Funny how the symptoms of a shedding uterus and one bulking up as an early home can so closely mimic each other.

Reflecting back, I knew. I knew that pulling out hadn't worked. I think I was in 7th grade the first time it had been lectured to me that the move didn't count as safe contraception. Everyone knew that. I knew that. Still, I would wait a couple days for my period. People were always late, and there's a first time for everything. Those days were long and torturous.

It was my fault. We'd made a decision, and I acted in discord with it. Yes, Sam had participated, but I was the instigator. If I was indeed pregnant, it was a mess. A massive mess. We were happy and the boys were happy. Everyone slept through the night. Our three-bedroom house fit us perfectly. We were able to plan our weekends and genuinely enjoy excursions to the city, parks, and museums. Sure, we still had to pack massive bags for the day, but it was manageable and didn't constantly feel frenetic. I was exercising at least three times a week, and a good babysitter meant Sam and I had regained a social life with friends and enjoyed date nights. We wanted to travel, and we wanted to be fully present and invested in everything Mac and Carter did.

My emotions ranged from mad (at myself) and scared (to tell Sam) to sad (that I wasn't pleased about the possibility). It was easy to keep my thoughts and fears to myself because Sam hadn't followed up at all on what transpired that afternoon at the lake. It wasn't on his radar as a looming risk, and we had had protected interactions since. Simply put, it wasn't at the top of his mind.

Finally, on a day I was working from home, I took the test to confirm what I already knew. I sobbed and then threw up my breakfast. I cursed and then cried some more. As soon as Sam left for the office and after dropping the boys at preschool, I pulled up the list on my phone and started dialing. In my days of waiting to test, I had already looked up clinics in the area. This was new territory for me, and it felt really, really strange. There wasn't a Planned Parenthood anywhere close, but I did find a couple other "women's clinics."

I didn't process that I was taking fate into my own hands. My knee-jerk reactions were driven purely by a desire for control; I was protecting our happiness. My mind wasn't open to an unexpected, unscripted next chapter. Problem solving and taking care of business was what I did. I was able to schedule a mid-morning appointment and got right in the car. The boys were in school until 3 pm, allowing me enough time to get to the clinic, solve the problem, and be back home with time to spare. Yes, I was in a hurry. The best analogy I can think of is the five second rule: if you pick the dropped piece of food up off the floor within five seconds, it's not technically dirty and can be safely consumed. If I acted quickly enough on this matter, it would be as if it had never happened. It could be erased from history.

I was on autopilot for the 15-mile drive, not letting myself consider or feel anything. I had low expectations for what I would walk into at the clinic. The ambiance was about as expected. It was clean with minimal décor, the staff were courteous, and the whole scene made me extremely uncomfortable. I looked up from the clipboard sporadically as I completed the paperwork. I was leery of using my real name, in case of a data breach. This was not a medical encounter I wanted floating around in the ether. I used the first moniker that popped in my head.

I felt out of place. Not better than the other women in the vinyl armchairs, but different. Our races were mixed, and my age was definitely advanced. I wondered what each of their stories was, and I consciously stayed away from stereotypes and assumptions. I was there, too, and I couldn't bear to think of the stories they might have created about *me*. I was fair game even though I didn't feel like I fit the profile. I was a happily married, financially stable mother of two with no good reason other than fear, uncertainty, and dreaded change to not welcome the idea of another child into my life.

The nurse called, "Casey," and I rose quickly to follow her through the door to the dated and sterile exam room. I needed to keep moving, or I might have run back out the door. The nurse was respectful and professional. My walls were up, big time; I wasn't interested in any chitchat. Neither was she. She took my vitals, did another pregnancy test, and explained the need for an ultrasound. I hadn't expected the ultrasound, but it was required to date the pregnancy and confirm its placement. I was irritated by the unanticipated step and just wanted to get out of there.

I'd never had a vaginal ultrasound. She walked me through the procedure, beginning with the insertion of the dildo-like wand. She positioned the wand and looked around. In the silence, she moved the wand this way and that, all the while keeping her eyes carefully fixed on the monitor. After about 60 very long seconds, I had to ask. It seemed she was coming up empty. She described that it must have been too early to visualize the pregnancy "material." Another analogy came to me: one can take a Strep test too quickly, too early. You can actually have Strep, but if the bacteria aren't sufficiently colonized for collection and identification, an initial test will come back negative. I was being punished for my efficiency. She finished up, had me sit up and re-secure my gown, and said she'd be back with the doctor. Things weren't going according to plan, and time and space started to warp. I temporarily didn't know who or where I was, and my hands began to tingle.

I was startled back into the moment when the door creaked open and in walked a man who looked like he played a doctor on TV. He wore green scrubs under a long gown that tied at his waist. The thick-rimmed glasses are what I remember most distinctly. Creepy. He wore a surgical mask, although no procedure was to be performed. This was pre-pandemic, so the mask stood out as odd. Unable to read his face, my focus went immediately to his eyes, which were not warm. They felt impatient and without compassion. He explained curtly that there was nothing he could do to "help" me that day. Protocol was that they needed to see the pregnancy on ultrasound to ensure against an ectopic pregnancy, a very dangerous circumstance. He instructed me to return in 7-10 days for retesting. I asked if there was anything I could sign releasing them of liability if they would just dispense the meds to me that day. I received a very quick and firm negative response. There was no fight to be had. So, I left, without a magic pill to fix my conundrum.

I will forever be extraordinarily and humbly grateful for that day's broken momentum. I now consider it to have been divine intervention. I was moving so quickly, too quickly, for my own good, but I didn't realize it at the time. My intention was to take care of business, to reset my life back to the way I thought I wanted it. I would have, if I could have, taken care of it that day. That was my clear intention. That's what turns my stomach as I share. Thank goodness for my hastiness and thank goodness for the protocol. If I had waited a week and they saw the pregnancy on ultrasound, I may not have my JJ.

I lived with the high-magnitude secret for another week and waffled every day, as if it were my choice alone. How pompous of me. I don't remember if I prayed about it. Back then I wasn't so connected as I am today. If this happened today, I would be on my knees, praying loudly for guidance. But I doubt I prayed then, which is just another reason I am so massively appreciative of the intervention, the pause in my plan. I didn't even ask for help, and He still helped.

I always considered myself to be pro-choice, mostly in consideration of cases of the mother being somehow at risk or of the fetus being known to be unviable. However, I never expected that I would consider abortion for myself. There, I said it. Even after my plan at the clinic was halted, I researched how to end a pregnancy naturally. I took high doses of vitamin C for a few consecutive days based on something I'd read online. It didn't work. Again, thank goodness.

I continued to keep my secret and tried to act normal. I avoided too much one-on-one time with Sam over those days because I'm a really bad liar. I don't remember reaching a conscious decision to keep the pregnancy. However, one morning, I took another test (probably my 15th) and brought it out to Sam as if it were the first. I was shaking and crying, and his reaction was perfectly positive. We each shared a couple thoughts about fears and doubts, but overall, we never looked back or questioned. I needed a partner in this acceptance, and having Sam made an immediate difference. We quickly realized that our thinking about how many children we wanted had been limited. We couldn't have made the decision on our own to throw a wrench into the life we were so satisfied with. Still, I've never shared with Sam that I knew for a few days and didn't tell and that I had serious doubts. Doubts so serious they inspired unilateral action. I see now that my thinking (or lack thereof) was superficial, selfish, fear-based, and incomplete, and that I hadn't thought through the ramifications.

From there, I quickly came to terms with my state. I scheduled an appointment with my regular OB/Gyne and quickly embraced the pregnancy as an opportunity to do it differently the third time. I had changed in the three years since I'd had Carter. I wanted a more natural pregnancy and birth experience, focused on healthy eating and exercise. I indulged in supportive resources and had a really beautiful pregnancy. We involved Mac and Carter with preparations at the house, and guess what? They were excited to share a room. Sam and I liked knowing our babies' sex in advance. There were enough surprises on delivery day, and our experience was that learning boy or girl was always as exciting as learning that we were pregnant in the first place. We took the boys to the 20-week ultrasound. The baby was happening to all of us, and we wanted them to feel engaged. At that point, I was scared it would be a girl. Practically, I didn't want princess castles next to trucks and sports balls on the toy room shelves. More emotionally, I worried that I wouldn't know what to do with a girl. I wasn't a high-maintenance female, and the drama of the preteen years terrified me. I sighed audibly when the ultrasound technician pointed at the boy parts. I adamantly believe that we're given what we're supposed to have, as it relates to children and life in general.

I was more physically and emotionally prepared for JJ's arrival than for my first two. It was a beautiful birth experience; one I would wish for all mothers. Mac and Carter came to the hospital in their "Big Brother" t-shirts and our party of five instantly felt right. Since I met him, JJ and I have been soulfully connected. It's safe to say that we have been deeply in love ever since. JJ was the only one of my three children I successfully breastfed. I needed him. I didn't know it, but someone else did. God, The Universe, The Higher Power, however you might refer to "it." I believe that JJ chose me as his mother. We are meant to be together in this life, this world.

For years now, I have offered prayers of thanks for my boys, especially JJ. I've never told another person that I nearly stopped his life. I may never tell Sam. I think he would be furious that I would have/could have thought the decision was mine alone. I can't imagine life without JJ. He's definitely my angel baby. I've considered at many points what life would have been like without him. The images are incomplete, lacking, and unfulfilled.

I've harbored guilt on many levels for years now. It's not fair that I didn't tell Sam right away. It was his clump of cells, too. I realize if I had managed to end the pregnancy that day that, although efficient, I never would have been able to sweep it under the rug and un-remember it the way I thought was possible. I don't think our marriage could have sustained the presence of that lie.

And perhaps even more significant, I've felt guilty on behalf of JJ. I didn't initially. It wasn't that when he was handed to me, I immediately felt unworthy. Instead, guilt has presented itself at random and unpredictable times, especially when I think about how blessed I've been with this immaculate child when I didn't initially believe I wanted him. That, when so many women would do anything to have a child at all. I have, at times, believed I'm monstrous, atrocious, and downright terrible. The guilt has been heavy. On this page, I hereby forgive myself once and for all and will forever embrace the glorious gift of JJ.

This is a story of being saved from myself and of someone, some force knowing better than me. It is not meant to share my thoughts on abortion or women's rights, nor to influence anyone else's. Not at all. That's your business, your destiny. I simply wanted to share my story in case it resonates with anyone else. This is to say that learning of a pregnancy—and becoming a mother—is no uncomplicated matter. I hear you and see you, and I want to encourage you to share your thoughts with someone, anyone. And by the way, doing so anonymously very much counts. It's okay to question. Please know you aren't alone.

Chapter 11

Flow

AMANDA

> "Someone told me to dream bigger, and I said, 'This is my biggest dream right now.' Just here to let you know that you get to decide what your big dream is."
>
> —Neha Ruch

I called Harmony House Academy, one of the top childcare choices in Boulder, early in my pregnancy with our first daughter. It felt premature, like we might jinx something, especially given my prior miscarriage. But word on the street was that we needed to get on the waiting list early. First availability for a visit was four months later, and Lane and I were one of five couples on the coveted 9 am Friday tour.

The receptionist's affable welcome, light-filled hallways lined with vibrant artwork, and giggling children all radiated warmth. Security cameras, scents of freshly cleaned spaces, and framed accreditation certificates promised safety. My mind checked the boxes as my heart's antennae scanned for the meaningful facts, the kind that inform decisions. Would our baby girl be nurtured and cherished there, in her hours away from us? Would she feel content and in community? Her early socialization was high on my list of priorities and an impetus for pursuing daycare in the midst of a global pandemic.

Perky Peggy paraded us past color-coded toddler classrooms, imaginative playscapes, and endless cubbies. She ticked off a list of morning procedures: change outdoor shoes to indoor shoes, sit around the ellipse taped to the floor for attendance and current events, and work with a partner on the day's first lesson. Having studied elementary education in college, I held a special appreciation for the systematic approach to caring for a large population of very young children. But still, I couldn't process all the details quickly enough. How would I know for sure if Harmony House was the right place for my baby? I would return as many times as necessary to feel comfortable and would build a spreadsheet of programming options, faculty credentials, and facility features, of course.

The last stop on the tour was the nursery, clearly the facility's pride and joy—the nest representing the bright beginnings of a fledgling's development at Harmony House. The room was spacious and bright, and the caregivers were very nurturing.

"Are you alright?" Lane asked.

I stood frozen, victim to the hurricane in my head.

"Amanda, I said, are you alright?" Lane repeated.

"Look at *all* those cribs," I said.

"That's a lot of babies. Amazing how quiet it is. And look at all those buggies over there. Do you think they take them all out at the same time? Impressive operation."

I pictured pumping, packing up enough bottles for the day (plus two extra), and handing my baby over to an 18-year-old to feed her. What if the bottles got mixed up in the industrial refrigerator, and she was fed another woman's milk in the unupholstered rocking chair? What if the room was too bright and she couldn't sleep? What if she fussed but no one heard her above other babies' cries? What if, what if, what if? Everything I knew about calming breath from my years as a yoga instructor went out the window. My mind's top-ranked futurization skills did not disappoint. I forced myself back to the moment. Daycare was what parents did. It was how people like us could take care of their babies and stay gainfully employed in order to pay the rent and buy healthcare insurance, all while making the most of their time with Baby in the morning and evening. It was the only option that made sense, and we had to jump on it.

After a detailed explanation of Harmony House's differentiated 1:2 caregiver to baby ratio, Peggy began to close out the orientation session. I discreetly eyed our peer parents-to-be, wondering what competitive advantages they may hold over us in having an admission application accepted. Did they know someone in Administration? Would they add another zip code to the attractively diverse client base? Did they have multiple children? What if they got in and we didn't?

Another of the expectant mothers asked the million-dollar question.

"I'll be returning to work in July," she said. "Will I be able to sign a contract to enroll mid-July?"

"Right now, we're taking applications for a year from June," Peggy said.

"Oh, thank God," I blurted under my breath.

There was no room at the inn, no place for my baby there. I pulled Lane toward the exit, diverting the group's attention. Turns out it was an alarmed emergency exit. Our walk turned into a run.

"Holy sh*t," Lane said in the parking lot. "Are you alright? You're scaring me."

"I can't put my finger on it. I panicked, I guess. All the babies were so well taken care of, and I know a ton of people who absolutely rave about this place."

"I'm not surprised," Lane said. "I never thought you'd be able to let someone else take care of your baby. I just came because you made me."

"So, what are we going to do?"

I was off the hook with Harmony House, a perfectly beautiful establishment. The glitch was that we didn't have other options, and I was due in six weeks. Hiring a nanny and having someone else in the house wasn't of interest. My parents were still working, my father the police chief in Estes Park and my mother a medical insurance coordinator after having been in law enforcement for years herself. Lane's parents were two and a half hours away in the mountains. They all would have been thrilled to help out, but it just wasn't a possibility.

Unsettled by the conundrum of who would take care of our baby and in need of a plan, we turned our options over every which way and eventually concluded that we would take advantage of the unique circumstances of COVID-19. We both worked entirely from home: I was in sales for a healthcare company, and Lane was a software engineer for a social media company. We figured we'd stagger our calls and juggle baby duties during business hours. We'd be creative and somehow make it work. Skepticism aside, that plan felt closer to making sense than daycare did to me. With that major decision made, we went on to enjoy my last trimester. I was bursting with energy those last weeks. We took road trips with Finn, our beloved Golden Retriever and our first baby. We loved on him hard in anticipation of soon needing to bide our attention.

Don't let anyone tell you that the nesting instinct isn't a real phenomenon. While we women may each experience it differently, it is very, very real. First, I'd change the sheets, just in case, and even if I'd changed them the day before. Then, I'd clean. Each day, a different room. Top to bottom, crevice to crevice. I was way beyond dusting and organizing. In the three weeks ahead of my due date, my fingertips were sore from scrubbing bathroom tile and grout. I wondered what passersby thought as I vacuumed the concrete walkway out front and hosed down the porch. I was large and in charge. I couldn't stop, and it wasn't because the former Marine sergeant I lived with was issuing orders. In fact, Lane tried to stop me when he found me alphabetizing our DVD collection in the middle of the night. Yes, we still have DVDs. I'd wake up each morning and do it all again.

My water broke an hour or two after going to bed on Lane's birthday, 17 days early. Pretty sure I hadn't peed myself (not out of the question at nine months pregnant), we mobilized. My mother had arrived in town earlier in the day, so I felt like less of a traitor leaving Finn with her. I vacuumed, took out the trash, and cuddled with Finn for a bit before heading to the hospital around 3 am. I was eight and a half centimeters dilated upon arrival and was told we would most likely be meeting our baby girl later that same day. That threw me for a loop, as I'd assumed she would be out momentarily. For as planful and prepared as I am, I had chosen not to spend much time researching childbirth because I didn't want to be scared. I quickly opted for an epidural, and after only a few pushes, there was Ava Lane in my arms 12 hours after my water broke. Efficient, if I do say. Lane and I basked in her flawlessness. Her hair felt like the silk of a fine scarf, and her complexion was as delicate as a flower's petal. Initial fawning complete, her perfection was confirmed. I texted my manager and VP of Sales to let them know of my status change and that I'd be sure to wrap up my outstanding work as soon as we arrived home. They didn't seem concerned.

Early nursing sessions were awkward, between the intense uterine cramping and twisting my body so Ava was comfortable. Plus, my mind was simultaneously composing emails to clients explaining my early departure. Just because I'd had a baby didn't mean I could skirt my professional responsibilities. I loved my job and clients, and I would not abandon them. I've been accused of caring too much, but I stand by my diligence. I transitioned every client to a back-up resource for the next 12 weeks, closed my laptop, and set my focus entirely on the one who needed me most.

Ava truly was an angel baby, crying only in the most justified circumstances. While no one is immune to the effects of sleep deprivation, my transition to a brand-new title was quite smooth. "Mommy" came naturally to me. After navigating a few breastfeeding bumps in the road, we hit our stride, and Ava thrived in every way. I always knew growing up that I wanted to have children, and so my healthy pregnancy and Ava's safe arrival following the miscarriage hit me hard as the grandest gift of my life. My dream was fulfilled. Beyond having a healthy baby, I didn't have a specific vision of my own motherhood, and I figured I'd do it the way those around me had. I cherished Ava in a way that was new to me, a way difficult to assign words to. I realize most mothers claim the same, yet the intensity of the devotion was incomparable to anything I had ever experienced. Maybe that's why I had such a hard time sharing her.

My mother stayed with us for several weeks, as she was living in Missouri at the time, and Lane's parents were with us for two days as well. So, in addition to my physical recovery, learning to care for my new jewel, and repeatedly repelling work thoughts from my mind, I was a bed-and-breakfast proprietor. I didn't know how to say "no" to visitors in those early weeks, so the house was always active, a revolving door. I scribbled a big mental note-to-self: the chaos of a full house on top of my need for order did not add up to an ideal postpartum landscape, at least for me.

Terrified a family member or run-of-the-mill visitor would drop Ava or deposit a germ in her sphere, I was grateful for her pokey eating. I stole away with her for feedings and private cuddles at every opportunity, regardless of who was in attendance.

As someone who is almost always in motion, I was awed by the joy and satisfaction of sitting perfectly still with her. Time and every other priority should have stopped as I drank in her sweet scent and smiling blue eyes (which she didn't get from me *or* Lane). Yet, even in those early days, my mind couldn't stay put. My impending return to work poked at me. How would I be okay with giving her any less than my full attention? I didn't let myself dwell and reminded myself of two things: 1) My great fortune in having Ava, period, and 2) Lane and I had a plan.

From the time she was a few weeks old, Lane and I alternated shifts in the early morning so the other could workout. The need for rigorous exercise is something Lane and I have always shared. So, as we entered parenthood, we were committed to protecting that sacred part of our individual and joint lives. The reinstatement of my 5 am workout routine was paramount to my ability to sustain energy despite little sleep.

In short, Lane and I made the most of our paternity and maternity leaves and thoroughly enjoyed our time bonding with Ava, nurturing the relationship between her and Finn, and taking family walks. We'd walk for miles fantasizing about the future. Always suckers for real estate open houses, we even walked through a few new-construction home sites and both fell in love with a cozy four-bedroom modern farmhouse. *#dreamers*

After 12 weeks, both of us returned to work with very full hearts. My heart was full, but my stomach was sour. I don't think I could have returned to a real office. The women who do are my heroes. The pandemic devastated many families. I will always honor that and will never minimize the lives lost. At the same time, I will also always recognize the gift COVID gave to our new family, the gift of working from home. Our plan to coordinate work calendars so that one of us was always with her while Ava was awake worked well initially because she was a rockstar napper.

Most everyone has a crawl-under-the-table with embarrassment virtual meeting story of glimpsing a coworker in a bathrobe, or worse. Always double, triple, quadruple checking that my computer camera was turned off, I pumped while on internal calls, enabling Lane to feed Ava when I wasn't available. On the surface, all was well. Ava chugged the homemade recipe, and Lane enjoyed the opportunity to feed her. I, however, quickly came to resent the pump, silicone, and meetings that kept me from the tiny human I made from scratch. I caught myself sounding chippy with clients and co-workers a couple of times, and that wasn't me. I'd always enjoyed and respected my teammates, but I had new difficulty participating in weather and sports-related small talk. 100% client satisfaction was my standard, but meetings with my hospital accounts and even discussions about patient safety began to feel trite. My strife in performing well across two disparate and major sets of responsibilities swelled. I checked myself daily to ensure my battle wasn't evident to those who mattered.

I didn't let up, and my work didn't suffer. Ava didn't suffer either; Lane or I was always there for her. Our arrangement worked for about a year. As she became mobile, it was more difficult to effectively play house *and* work professionally. I was the one who suffered. I was on a neighborhood moms text string, so I knew about the meetups at the park on Tuesdays and Thursdays when I had standing client check-ins. Parent-infant story time at the library was mid-morning when I definitely needed to be at my computer. If I did walk away from my desk before 5 pm to be with Ava, I felt tremendous guilt. I stuffed the sadness and told myself how lucky I was to have a work-at-home scenario and a hands-on husband. I pressed on. I couldn't tell Lane that I wanted to be a stay-at-home mom because I didn't exactly realize it myself. As soon as the idea flickered in my mind, I reminded myself that our life was predicated on dual income and that a gap in my work history would penalize me in the future. Also, it wasn't the 1950's.

My mother worked, and so would I. My friends with babies worked; they did it all, and I would too. I wasn't a quitter and wasn't about to become one. As vaccines became readily available and the threat of a return to business travel loomed, I blocked it out. There was no way in the world I would leave Ava. I would deal with it when I had to. And I would indeed have to, if we were really going to engage the outlandish idea of purchasing that farmhouse. Lane and I have always made quick (not hasty!) decisions, the timing of which didn't always make obvious sense. We couldn't get the house out of our minds, couldn't shake the deep knowing that it was meant to be ours. I wanted the house, but that also meant I needed my job.

I expected that, in motherhood, I would be better able to avoid working after hours, but that didn't pan out. It was impossible to compartmentalize work from personal correspondence on my phone. For me, looking was better than wondering what might be lurking in my inbox. My incessant checking of emails became an unconscious behavior akin to a nervous twitch, and I wasn't good at leaving to-dos for later. At the end of each day, I justified my attention to my phone and computer with the knowledge that Ava wouldn't remember my diverted gaze. I felt guilty not giving her my complete attention, and I felt like a bad employee for my fragmented workdays. Completing everything on both my domestic and professional lists didn't equate to feeling accomplished. I woke up early each day and did it all again.

Once Ava started sleeping later in the morning, Lane and I could work out together, which was our favorite kind of date. On a typical morning, I could sneak in five miles on the treadmill before showering to be ready to make Ava breakfast and spend a little time together before work. I had a bad habit of scrolling through emails while striding. It was not only a safety hazard but also made staying in the present moment impossible. It turns out that it also poses a risk of self-realization. The volume of emails that morning wasn't the problem; it was their content, including an RFP (request for proposal) from a major health system. I made the mistake of opening the attachment and taking a precursory look through the bazillions of questions. My feet got heavy, and my ankles felt wobbly. My appropriately exerted breathing morphed into panicked, shallow, ineffective gasps for air that led to tearful squawks. My vision blurred.

Deep into his squat circuit and through his noise cancelling AirPods, Lane heard my shrieks and hurried over.

"Honey, what is it?" he begged. "Did someone die or something?"

I've never been a crier, so what else could be going so wrong before 6 am? I continued to run.

"Amanda, what is it?" he raised his voice.

"An RFP," I managed through the tears that were falling into and out of my mouth.

"Please stop running," he pleaded. "This isn't safe. Get off!"

As my arms and legs flailed, I disregarded the treadmill's red safety key. Devoid of my poise on the yoga mat, I flew off the belt, landing in a pile at the end of the machine.

"Sorry, I don't understand," Lane said kneeling next to me, now that he knew no one was dead. "You do RFPs all the time, and you win most of them."

I couldn't put into words the epiphany that had just shot through me like a super-charged bolt of lightning. I struggled to make sense of it myself. I was heaving heavily at that point, unable to vocalize at all.

"Why don't you go walk around the block, cool down," he suggested lightly. "I'll get Ava up and feed her. Then we can talk."

I nodded.

"You're not hurt, right?" Lane asked before leaving the scene. I shook my head as if it were attached by a string of dental floss, still mute.

Composing myself took a little time, even after I was dressed. I found my words and mustered my courage to share the clarity that had come to me. Ava enjoyed a cup of dry cereal and an episode of Sesame Street while we talked.

"Here's the thing. Not everyone gets to be a mother," I said. "I was given this tremendous gift, and I want every second with Ava. Every hour I'm not with her, I'm miserable. The time is already slipping away, and I really just don't want to work anymore. There, I said it."

"That's it? That's all?" he asked, reaching for my hand. "Honey, if this is that big of a thing, quit your job. We'll figure it out."

"Really?" I asked, burying my head in his chest and crying again, this time tears of joy. "Really, you mean it? I promise I'll go back before too long if I can just have this time with Ava now."

Immediate relief engulfed me as soon as I said it out loud. My fall from grace wasn't really about the RFP, of course. The 50-page report was simply the final straw, shining a glaring light on the fact that something about the way I was living was misaligned. I was living according to what I had seen others do and the assumptions I had made. I hadn't wanted to let myself, Lane, or my hardworking parents down. Yet, I could no longer ignore that the arrangement wasn't working for me. Others saw the discord in me before I saw it in myself.

The conversation with Lane was easy, as they typically are. He has always been supportive of me. My primary concern was financial, but with some adjustments, it looked like we would be able to swing it on Lane's salary for a while. We would have to forego the idea of moving, but I didn't care if it meant I could be with Ava. There were subsequent conversations to get through, and I worried that they might not go as smoothly. First, we had my parents over for dinner, which was good practice speaking my newly realized truth.

"I have something to tell you that'll be a big surprise," I began. "It surprised me too, but nothing has been the same since I had Ava."

"What is it, dear?" Mom asked. "I can't imagine what you're going to say. Are you pregnant?"

"Ha, no. We're going to be making a change that I hope you can understand," I went on. "I really love my job, but I love Ava more and want to be with her every second I can. I've decided to stop working for a while."

"Amanda, my darling," Dad said. "I'm surprised it's taken you this long. Your mom and I have both thought that your paycheck job isn't where your heart is."

Their support and love were so clear that I didn't know where to look. "I was so scared you'd be disappointed," I said. "Both of you have had such impactful careers."

My mom went on for a few minutes, reiterating that we each get to choose how we pursue motherhood and that the beauty of it is that we get to keep choosing over and over again. I was heartened to discover her perspective, considering her own uninterrupted career.

Just the glimpse of my forthcoming freedom to serve Ava exclusively fueled me to see the RFP through . . . and win it. I resigned quickly thereafter. My managers were ever gracious, basically promising me my job back at any time. These affirmations told me it was alright to honor my current dream, unanticipated as it was, and that there *would* be a path forward. I chose to accept, rather than fight, that I didn't find peace in the intersection of my two jobs.

Once I resigned, it took my brain some time to adjust, to cease the cycling and constant auditing it was accustomed to.

I was instantly happier. Our days were never dull; I soaked in every book we read, every outing to the park, and every meal I fed Ava. I relished that she could count on me always and completely. The financial sacrifices for me to be home have been easy to make. We rarely eat out and instead enjoy the challenge of pursuing healthier options and making meals together at home. We cut the travel budget, reducing big trips to every two or three years. Fortunately for us, both sets of our parents live in beautiful places. We enjoy our escapes to these free-lodging destinations. Shopping trips are fewer, as are visits to the salon, but I have never questioned my decision or felt slighted in the least bit. The stars aligned, and our house sold for more than asking, enabling us to just barely cinch our dream house. Stretch goals!

We welcomed our second daughter, Zoe Jade, when Ava was about two and a half years old and following another miscarriage. Growing up, I always told my dad that I was going to name my children in the order of the alphabet. After having one and realizing that 26 children would be too many, I knew the name of our second angel had to begin with "Z." Our babies who came to us but couldn't stay taught me how to practice endurance and resilience when chasing dreams. They are always here with us and are part of the backdrop of my immense gratitude for Ava and Zoe. They will always be my first "A" and "Z." Mommy loves you.

Being a stay-at-home mom cast a completely different light on my pregnancy, delivery, and postpartum experience with Zoe. I vividly recall Lane bringing Ava to the hospital to meet her baby sister. Holding Zoe and with Ava on the bed between my legs, it registered that "it's us three girls now." It was a holy moment. My attention was pure, unadulterated. There were no distractions this time. No boss or clients to email, no back-up utility to call in. My transition with Zoe was far superior because my mind wasn't doing mental gymnastics. This time we limited visitors and protected our private family time. There was no looming return to work in 12 weeks or the daunting call to talk to Lane about my conflicted heart—such a breath of fresh air. This time around with Zoe, I haven't pumped once. I'm not overtly trying to keep her from Lane, but I do love that I'm the only one who can feed her. This is part of my dream.

As I nursed Zoe one afternoon, no screens were in sight, our eyes locked, and my mind wandered to yoga's core tenets. The mind-body connection and the concept of flow have always intrigued me, despite my track record of not being very good at "going with the flow." My process of pivoting to stay-at-home motherhood honed my recognition that the Universe moves through everything. Like a river's current, nothing stays exactly the same; everything changes in a good way, allowing for fresh expression. I recently read a blogger's description of the flow of the Universe. The author described the Universe's flow as rocks that form, get pounded into dust, and are blown away. For me, it's the sprouting of a summer flower born from a seed planted in the spring. It's the growth cycle of every human. Flow is the current that carries us down our life's path. When we move with the flow rather than resist it, we are moving in the way that is intended for us. Our flow is unique, just like our fingerprints, which means that the paths of others aren't necessarily relevant to our own path. Because forever is a long time, I am committed to at least temporarily letting go of the notion that I need to be in control of all things at all times. Rather, I control what I can (reasonably) and then take the ride.

While my days are now hard in different ways, I'm no longer conflicted. My time and mind are still very busy, but they are harmonized and streamlined entirely around the girls' needs, desires, and schedules. It feels so right. But that doesn't mean I don't experience gremlins or miss things about my paid position.

You should be working. What am I setting myself up for in the future? How am I going to get back into the workplace? I miss the exhilaration of business presentations and the stress of deadlines. I miss solving a complicated business problem, and I miss my sales team. But I have a new team now, and I love being captain for Ava and Zoe. I very intentionally don't have a five-year plan. Instead, I have faith that answers to the questions of the future will present when they need to.

I will forever be grateful for my breakdown on the treadmill. It awakened me to no longer just *wish* things were different, and it inspired me to *make* things different. I was shown what I couldn't see by applying logic alone. It forced me to be brave in order to save myself. I surrendered to going with the flow without realizing it, and I honored my dream I hadn't seen coming. Thinking back to our tour of Harmony House Academy, there was nothing at all wrong with the place. It was a beautiful environment. It just wasn't aligned with my not-yet-conscious resistance to letting someone else take care of my baby. From the vantage point of today, I can recognize my budding dream to take care of Ava myself. I didn't want to share her. I see how flow is always taking us where we need to go. It's only a matter of whether we take the ride or drag our feet.

I've learned that how I do life and how I do motherhood isn't up to anyone or anything but me. It's not up to my parents and how they did things, it's not up to my friends and what fulfills them, it's definitely not up to society, and it's not even up to Lane. I am blessed with a partner who sees me and loves me for who I am, which is currently a mother who loves fiercely.

Whatever is on your heart and whatever is right *for you* will always be the right decision. It doesn't need to make sense to someone else. There is always an opportunity to change your path along the way. Who knows, I could be pulling my hair out in two years and be screaming, "Get me back to the office." No decision is final; nothing is permanent. Even dreams change. They are meant to change according to the flow.

And so, I say, "Namaste." I bow to you. The light in me sees, honors, and loves the light in you. Let's do our best to shed the layers of what and whom we think we are and keep shedding until we arrive at our true essence, our true self. Let's be patient and gentle with ourselves because it's challenging when the target of truth is steadily evolving. Let's love the current version of ourselves, our "now" selves. And let's not be as surprised as I was when future versions find us. Let's be open and love them, just as we do our past selves. Let's flow together.

Chapter 12

Red Rope

ASHLEE

"Let choice whisper in your ear and love murmur in your heart. Be ready. Here comes life."
—Maya Angelou

I didn't know there was such a thing as being too happy, but I've been accused of the condition. As a homebuilder, I've had an occasional client question my excessive happiness, and one actually requested to work with a colleague of mine instead. I don't get it, but to each her own. Those who embrace my happiness tell me I'm a beacon of positivity. Not the inspirational quote kind of positivity that temporarily boosts our mood but doesn't withstand the tough stuff. I'm talking about the inherent positivity I hold within and that governs my whole being and all my choices. The kind of positivity that's the foundation for resilience when life doesn't go according to plan.

Josh and I were newlyweds and fully engaged in all that entails. I was a real estate agent, and Josh had recently finished chiropractic school and was establishing his new practice. We were also intent on establishing a family. As the oldest of 13 children,

I'd been a mother for as long as I could remember and was ready to have a baby of my own. We were elated to be pregnant for the second time, but my file was flagged. History of a previous miscarriage meant a comprehensive ultrasound at 18 weeks instead of 20. I'd attended many ultrasounds with my mom, so I knew mine was taking too long. Something wasn't right. I looked at Josh; he didn't look fazed. But I was.

The ultrasound tech wasn't at liberty to tell us what she saw—or didn't see—and summoned Dr. Paquette, my OB.

"There are some brain formations we need to get a closer look at," Dr. Paquette explained. "We'll get you over for an MRI today to understand if there's anything to be concerned about."

When she called with the scan results, I was driving down Hawaii Street, the Minnesotan sun pelting my windshield.

"Ashlee, your baby has Holoprosencephaly," she said.

"Holo, what?" There aren't many seven-syllable words in our language.

She spelled it out, and I frantically wrote it in my hand because I couldn't find any paper in the car.

"The anatomy of his brain is compromised," she explained. "The right and left hemispheres aren't separated like they should be."

"So I'm having a boy?" I slurred through the lump in my throat, focusing on what I understood.

"Yes, your baby's a boy, Ashlee."

Dr. Paquette described the problems associated with the two sides of his brain not properly communicating. A wide range of physical and neurological deficits would present symptoms of unpredictable severity. From the get-go, there were many more unknowns than there were certainties. How long would he live? If he did live, what would his quality of life be? What would our lives be like as the parents of a special needs child?

"Please don't Google it," Dr. Paquette urged. "You'll find lots of things that go against hope. The information could be scary. Your baby will write his story, and we'll focus on that."

I gave myself a moment and honored the devastating news with a long, hard cry. Then, against Dr. Paquette's advice, I started my research. Babies with holoprosencephaly are often stillborn or die shortly after birth. The 3% who do survive birth are commonly born with a cleft lip or palate, some without a nose, or with one eye (cyclopia). Others don't have a stomach. I proceeded to cry for two weeks and dodged my friends' innocent and supportive inquiries about the ultrasound. "Did you see the tiny toes?" "Is it a girl? A boy?"

Following batteries of additional tests, we learned that our baby's specific diagnosis was of moderate severity—semi-lobar holoprosencephaly, which didn't help to clarify his future. Would he live for minutes, months, or more? I swam in the unfathomable question of what life would be like. Most specifically, what it would be like for him. *Is this what mothers do? Bring their children into the world to suffer?* My Christian upbringing said abortion was wrong, period, end of story. Geneticists presented us with grim diagnostic reports and statistics right along with our options to terminate. It was a classic battle of faith vs. facts, and logic could only get us so far. My whole life was in turmoil. I didn't know what it all meant or what to do, and no one could tell me. Competing voices echoed loudly in my head, taking advantage of my especially tender state.

Josh and I were aligned, but as my baby's mother, I was the only one who could make this choice. I was invaded by messaging that I wasn't enough, that he'd suffer, and that he would have no meaningful quality of life. While I was always inclined to keep the pregnancy, I needed guidance beyond my own thoughts. I brought the decision to God. In prayer, I closed my eyes, shut out the noise all around me, and asked God for a clear answer. I could feel my soul shaking, and a knowing came over me. The message was clear: there was something remarkable before us, a gift of the greatest proportions. It was a very real moment, processing the reality of what I was about to say yes to. Feelings of insufficiency were replaced with a wave of valor as Josh and I chose to support our baby boy the best we could. We named him Levi.

Spoiler alert: this is not a sad story. There are scary moments and sad happenings for sure, but on the whole, this is a story about my journey with a little boy who never said a word but touched people's hearts. A boy who never took a step but left footprints everywhere he went. In the eyes of the world, this child would be quickly dismissed, but each day, I watched as he inspired my transformation and that of others into who we should all be.

Once we'd confirmed our decision with the medical team, I had another choice to make; I could see the situation as something tragic, or I could see each day as a gift that never had to be. The world was going to be against him. How could I be anything but *for* him? I warrior-ed up and welcomed motherhood. I wasn't focused on how many moments and days there were to come; I focused only on the present moment. As long as we were together, I was his mother. His chances of surviving outside my body informed my acceptance that my pregnancy might be the extent of my motherhood, of our time together. Even if he didn't survive birth, we would have known each other and loved each other. I clung to hope that he'd defy the odds. I prepared a nursery against counsel to buy a casket, not a crib. The normalcy in nesting was so refreshing. I loved being pregnant and did everything in my power to nourish him physically and spiritually. Sometimes, that looked like adding a heaping dose of highly concentrated fish oil to my morning smoothie. I knew

DHA wasn't going to fix anything, but it was my way of giving him his best chance. Other times I patted my firm belly and prayed for a miracle.

The joyful anticipation of a new life always won out over the slippery slopes of fear and self-pity. I wanted to spread the joy, so I wrote a poem that Christmas. It was written as a message from Levi, and I included it with our holiday card. It began, "I'm not a normal baby, and I don't know what that means. I'm coming, and I'm not what you're expecting. I'm special . . ." Everyone knew I was pregnant, but not everyone knew his diagnosis. In my earliest advocacy for him, I wanted to share who was coming to get ahead of awkwardness at his arrival and beyond. People's questions, comments, and actions were mostly well-meaning, but they could still be uncomfortable. So, I wrote the poem as an act of generosity, a practical favor, an emotional preparation for who and what was to arrive in February. I focused on protecting him and on recruiting our troops of support.

My physical pregnancy was relatively easy until about 30 weeks, when I developed preeclampsia. We were both monitored closely, and by 37 weeks, my elevated blood pressure and intensified swelling were of high concern, along with the increasingly imminent risk of seizures. Dr. Paquette strongly encouraged induction, and I agreed. My hope, tempered in reality, was that he'd come out breathing. He wanted to stay with me, so a lot of Pitocin was needed to coax him out. I delivered 8-pound Levi Joshua at the conclusion of a fairly normal labor and vaginal delivery. He came out breathing on his own and with a strong heart, both atypical for Holoprosencephaly babies. We were off to a promising start.

I gave birth at a standing-room-only show. The hospital room was filled with my parents, Josh's parents, and the magnanimous medical team. We knew the grandparents might only see Levi once, and we wanted to be together to baptize him. Little Levi was welcomed with infinite love, and in spite of my ultimate exposure in childbirth, it was a sacred moment to share. My epidural didn't work, so I was able to quickly get out of bed to see him as the team frantically conducted their initial assessments over in the corner. I needed to be at his side. I was desperate to touch him but didn't dare invade the gaggle of hands, cords, and tubes.

"Hon, it's our little surfer dude," I smiled as Josh held me up on the periphery of the team's huddle. "His hair's even longer than it looked in the ultrasounds."

His hair was all I took in before Levi was hurried away to the NICU. Our newfound physical separation throbbed everywhere within me, especially knowing he might not make it. The complicated pregnancy and highly emotional start to our next chapter caught up with me. I staggered, barely making it back to the bed to deliver a deteriorated placenta. My hemorrhaging and volatile vitals necessitated an emergency D&C. That night was humbling and so vulnerable. I was entirely depleted and had nothing left, including my baby, who had been taken from me.

As soon as I was intact, Josh raced my wheelchair to the buzzing NICU. Two nurses backed away from Levi's isolette, making room for us to adore our sweet boy. He had microencephaly (a small head), his hormones were way out of whack, and he didn't have an anal opening. One of his eye sockets was undersized and didn't open. I like to say he came out winking at me, heralding, "We're good, Mom, we got this." Levi's affirmation wore off all too quickly.

Reports of problem after problem continued, some more acutely life-threatening than others. The first of several surgeries we weren't sure he'd survive was his colostomy at only three hours old. Truth be told, I didn't know what a colostomy was. My first reference was to a colonoscopy. I was 22 and didn't have a dictionary of gastro-intestinal terms in my head. Even so, I was Levi's chief advocate, and I learned as I went. I didn't spontaneously defer but instead took the time to understand what the doctors said needed to happen, along with the ramifications of following (or not following) their directives. The colostomy wasn't much of a choice; he would die quickly without the procedure. Understanding was one thing, but it wasn't everything. That was my first beautiful lesson in trust, trusting the doctors. I visualized white light around us, practiced ultimate vulnerability, and surrendered Levi's life to the team as I handed him over.

My first diaper change involved a PICU nurse teaching me how to place a wafer, or skin barrier, over Levi's stoma. A stoma is a surgical procedure that secures the intestine in such a way that it protrudes through the abdomen in order to adhere to a colostomy bag for the collection of stool. In theory, no poopy diapers seemed like a decent trade. But as wafers blew off and lost their tackiness, the ordeal proved to be a challenge. Containing a bacterial frenzy and keeping it clear of a feeding tube centimeters away was a lot for a two-day-old mother. My adrenaline didn't diminish, and I eagerly learned the nuances of caring for Levi and his physical differences.

The monitoring of my own postpartum state fell under the radar as the spotlight shone on Levi. I was a post-op patient myself, battling the aftermath of preeclampsia and a D&C. I didn't feel well. I couldn't tell anyone because I'd be forced to leave Levi, so I stayed silent. The physical and emotional throes of postpartum are no joke for any new mother, regardless of the details of pregnancy, birth, and Baby's health. Mine escalated: my uterus was mad, clamping down on itself every few minutes. Headaches ensued, and my vision began to blur. I became nauseous. All the things they warned me could be serious side effects of preeclampsia following delivery were happening. Like a Pfizer Pharmaceuticals ad, thoughts of "may cause stroke or even death" reverberated in my head.

In the words of Viktor Frankl, "When we have a who, we can bear almost any how." I didn't know how I was going to get through, but I did know there was a who that needed me. I pressed on despite the warning signs.

"Keep pumping, Mama; he needs it," the nurses said.

I wiped sweat from my forehead, although I was moving at a snail's pace. Blood between my legs, the stress of pumping, and my oozing hormones had me haggard, but none of that mattered. I was on a mission to keep my son alive, and no one was coming around to fluff my pillow or inquire about me anymore. I couldn't remember when I'd last showered, and it was starting to feel like something that needed to happen. Once I knew Levi was stable, I grabbed a towel and washcloth from the nursing station.

Weak as I was, I grasped the hallway rail and hobbled to the public shower room. The corners were pinking, and the dispensers were empty and broken. Untended, perhaps it was used only in desperate times like mine. I turned the water on, sat on the stool, and peeled my clothes off. I stepped onto the frigid tile on the tips of my toes. Water fell on my head and down my face, and as if the weight of the drops was too heavy to carry, I collapsed. My left cheek lay in a pool of water against the cold penny tile floor, and blood veined through the water, collecting around the obstructed drain. Falling streams of water bounced off my limp body and into my eyes, further blurring my vision. For a split second, I was trapped inside a lifeless frame. I squinted my eyes and scanned the surroundings for the red rope. You know, that red emergency cord in literally every room in a hospital. Even if all you're doing is leaving a urine sample, there's a red rope. Every room has one. From the shower floor, I looked again. There was no red rope. There is no red rope for the mother.

I was alone, wet, cold, weak, and no one was coming for me. Worse yet, a sick little boy was depending on me for his life. I thought to myself, "If you don't get up, no one's going to take care of him. He needs you. You gotta get up, Ashlee."

My soul's strength gave my body energy. I managed to pull myself up to stand, desperately thumbed through the clothes I'd come in with, and got them back on my body. I glanced in the mirror at my white lips and fearful eyes. I was clinging to life. "I'll brush my teeth when I feel better," I thought. With one last glance at the girl in the mirror, I nodded as if to say goodbye. The girl I had been could only take me to that point. The girl who was newly required was the woman she'd become, the woman she could never have been without the girl in the mirror. I hugged her in my heart as I turned the doorknob to exit and made my way down the somber, dark hallway to save my son.

We brought Levi home from the hospital when he was one month old. While we were anxious to get our little family settled at home, I needed that time under the tutelage of the hospital nurses to learn my two new jobs. In addition to being a new mother, I'd earned an honorary nursing degree. Our house was converted to a MASH unit, a hospital: the fridge was stocked with saline bags and IV nutrition alongside produce and dairy products, and the linen closet doubled as storage for syringes, sterile dressings, and shelf-stable formula. Towels and bed sheets weren't at the top of my mind anyway. Despite having set up the nursery, Levi never stayed there. He always stayed with me in our bed, so I guess the nursery really was for me after all. I kept him with me so I could hear his heartbeat and put my hand under him. Feeling him breathe allowed me to sleep. His pulse-ox monitor's beep was my version of a white-noise machine, signaling to me that he was good and that I could let go, if only for a bit.

Finding community was difficult, and even if I could've gotten to a new moms group, it wouldn't have applied to me. Our existence was so wildly different, so foreign to most. I had oxygen and feeding tubes to contend with. I figured out how to wear a backpack and run the feeding tube through it so I could hold Levi close and feed him at the same time. I wasn't privy to the mother-to-mother connection that some get at the playground or coffee shop because I wasn't at those places. I weighed his output in the colostomy bag to know how much to feed him and how much IV fluid to give him, which is not exactly conducive to a societal setting. Caring for Levi was a constant chase, a race I ran gladly. But I wasn't a pro right away. We almost lost him when he was three months old, and he continued to have serious GI issues his entire life. If he had too much sensory input, he'd have what's called an Ileus, meaning his bowels would shut down, causing him to not eat for days, resulting in dehydration and hospitalization. I did find a few online connections and opportunities to chat about things like error readings on feeding pumps or brands of TPN (Total Parenteral IV Nutrition). Mostly, I was in it by myself. Josh helped when he was home, but he was trying to pay the bills. My parents couldn't be overly involved because they still had 10 kids themselves, and Josh's parents lived out of state.

Levi and I had a connection like I've never experienced, an unspoken language, a secret set of codes. We knew each other inside and out on physical, psychological, and spiritual levels. I could look into his eyes and understand, "Okay, I get it bud." I needed to titrate up three ccs on his IV. I lived in a state of constant adrenaline. As Mama Bear, I was always on the lookout for the next threat, and they were all around us. It could have been a tube, a hormone, a virus, anything. I saved his life over and over, sometimes multiple times a day. Like all moms, I kept my baby alive. It just looked a little—okay, a lot—different for us.

Believe it or not, I was rarely discouraged. I've always said to myself, "Ashlee, give the day your very best. And at the end of the day, if you can say you have indeed given it your best, then there are no regrets." That mantra got me through every day of my time with Levi. I always asked and challenged myself with "What's the next best thing I can do?" Some days, it was moment to moment like that all day long, and I drew so much strength from Levi himself. I believe we're all given the exactly right parents for us, and I know Levi came to me because I was going to say "yes" and embrace each challenge in exchange for the opportunity to grow in unforeseen capacities.

From the beginning, I knew that Levi wasn't his medical problems, and his problems didn't add up to who he was. He was the opposite of a problem; he was my greatest teacher, honing my gratitude for life's simple moments. Josh and I enjoyed many of the activities most parents enjoy. We read to him and sang lullabies at bedtime. He loved to swing, so we installed a swing in the kitchen ceiling. His smiles replenished us. The rumble strips on the side of the highway made him giggle, so we'd go driving. His laughter further filled us. He loved toys with dramatic lights. We put him in the right places and positions to experience life the best he could, and his contentment was our compass. Life with Levi wasn't easy, but it was rewarding, fulfilling, and full of so much love.

Josh and I felt strongly and actively that we had more love to give. Holoprosencephaly is hereditary, and the genetic mutation came from Josh's side. Still, we wanted more children. The doctors advised with 96% certainty that our subsequent children would have conditions as serious and life-threatening as Levi's. So, surrogacy, sperm donation, and adoption were suggested. We loved Levi like crazy, and we knew we would love anyone else who was given to us just as much. I realize that stance could be easily scoffed at. But when you've experienced the joy that comes from giving of yourself like I gave to Levi, the choice of "yes" comes easily. I believe that our two healthy biological children are God's reward to me for having trusted.

When Gianna was born a year and three months after Levi, I was grateful for every single healthy moment. Having grown up in a big family with babies all around me, I knew what every day parenting was. I took nothing for granted, and occasions like Gianna beginning to crawl meant so much more than checking a box. I knew such milestones weren't guaranteed. She came out a-blazin' and was opening cabinets at six months old and smashing my coffee pot on the tile floor at eight months. Have at it, Honey. Take the coffee pot! I sat and watched with awe. Gianna's baby dolls had central ports and feeding tubes. She'd syringe out and do all the things for her babies that I did with Levi. Her reality was different from that of most young children. We were aware of that and did everything in our power to cater to her and pay her the attention she so deserved.

I couldn't have done it without Theresa, our amazing PCA (personal care assistant) who took care of Levi during the day while I was a mom to Gianna. Theresa was and still is a member of our family, the best wing-woman I could ever have asked for. We juggled every day, and many balls dropped out of the air. But everyone was well cared for and more than amply loved. Eventually, Bennett joined the party to make the majority of the household male. I'm a different mother to Gianna and Bennett because I had the perspective of knowing that I might not be here forever. *They* might not be here forever. From a place of positivity, I continuously ask myself what I need to accomplish in the time I have with them. We knew we could lose Levi at any point, so we celebrated his birthday every month with over-the-top, miraculous salutes to the wisest teacher of my life. That's 64 birthdays and five years more than he was predicted to have.

With my encouragement, Josh and Gianna left town one weekend for a family reunion. So, it was only Levi, Bennett, and me at the house, a lighter load. I woke up before dawn to every alarm going off. Oxygen, food pump, everything. I had never slept through any alarm, not once. I looked over at Levi, and he was blue. The cannula had slipped out of his nose somehow. I picked him up, ripping the cords out of the wall, and called 911. My recollection from there is like something out of a movie, everything happening in slow motion. I brought Levi down the hall, and the EMTs met us in the foyer. Multiple people worked to revive him, pumping, prodding, and pleading. While they worked, I screamed. Wretched screams like I had not let out for five years. I didn't need to be strong anymore because he was gone, and I knew it.

Tears bellowed from my eyes as I knelt close to Levi, surrounded by medical personnel. I looked up, and my eyes focused on a beloved painting of Jesus, one hand on His heart and the other outstretched toward me. Beneath Him were the words, "Jesus, I trust in you." Jesus had him. I felt peace and told the team to stop, to let him be in Heaven. I picked up his lifeless body and pulled him close. No matter how tightly I held him, my soul wasn't satisfied because he wasn't there.

I believe God put me in a deep sleep that night and removed my family members who would have heard an alarm because He knew I would have fought really, really hard to keep Levi with me. But it was his time, and it wasn't mine to interfere with. I couldn't have made that choice.

Levi was a gift we knew we'd have to return too soon. His soul was the gift. His body was merely the package. I've never handed back a gift because I didn't like the wrapping. Levi was not a body that was broken but a carefully created soul given to me to tell a story. What a mighty story it was! Day in and day out, I loved his frail body the best I could so I could be with his soul a little bit longer. He guided me in knowing that his desire was the same. His bright eyes, his smiles, his giggles told me. Everything I gave to him physically for five years came back to me ten-fold in the person I've become. Who I am today would never be if I hadn't been Levi's mom first. No question. Who I am as a mother to living children, who I am as a wife, who I am in business, the leader I am, what I put out to the world—it's all different because Levi was here. The extent to which we feel suffering and pain is the extent to which we're made to feel joy. I believe that with all my heart, and I want to spread that joy. That's why *I'm* here.

Whether our children are healthy or facing medical challenges, under our roof or on their own, here on Earth or in Heaven, they are always with us. Once a mom, always a mom until the very end. Our babies' DNA remains in us, fragments having migrated in utero to our liver, thyroid, or other organs. Our children are literally always with us. Although I can't physically put my arms around Levi, my heart is always wrapped around him. I'm with him, and he's with me. The name Levi means "joined together," which I didn't learn until after he was gone. We were and always will be a beautiful team, yin and yang. Levi never had a voice, and I'm good at speaking. He couldn't write, and I'm a good writer. That wasn't by mistake. God doesn't make mistakes. Levi's sweet soul taught our family empathy: to open our hearts a little wider, love a little deeper, and give more of ourselves so we may radiate love and light.

Levi left this world nearly 10 years ago, and only recently have I grieved the losses associated with mothering him. It's as if I'm living our story for the first time as I heal because I didn't allow myself to feel the difficult emotions at the time. I was in survival mode and don't remember ever feeling negative. I admit that the stuffing of emotions shouldn't necessarily be emulated. While I faithfully did what needed to be done for Levi, *I* was becoming a new, elevated person. Today, I'm writing a book to invite people to heal as their stories are happening because life was hard knocks for me, and it doesn't need to be for you. You can start to see the world in a radically different way while the hardship is happening instead of waiting until it's over.

To mothers met with uncertain pregnancies, fretful diagnoses, and their children's suffering, these situations can rattle you, letting fear weave itself into every dream and threaten every happy thought. It's important to sit and face the reality of your moment. And at the same time, match fear with an equal amount of hope. Calming emotions allow us to peek at the beauty of what is before us and to dare to consider the transformation about to take place within us.

As mothers, we sacrifice ourselves for our children. It's a remarkable aspect of nature; it's the pelican move. A female pelican will beat her breast until it bleeds to feed her offspring. We mothers are immensely powerful beings, capable of incredible feats, bold intuition, and warrior-like protection, particularly when it comes to supporting our children.

Perhaps there will be a circumstance that greets you and asks you to be braver than you ever imagined possible. A circumstance that has you desperately searching for the red rope. I pray there's beautiful support wrapped around you in times of challenge. And yet, whether you have 10 people, two people, or no people coming to your aid, the story before you will create within you the person that you're here on Earth to become. You will experience the battles and the victories, and you will look back and realize that the strength you longed for in pulling the red rope, the hero you desperately desired, was the warrior within you waiting to rise through the ashes before you. Rise, warrior, rise! Everything you need is within.

Epilogue

Matrescence and Me

"*Let motherhood change you. Let it rearrange you. Let it soften your hard edges. Let it release your rules and rigidity. Let it unravel you. Let go. Let it go. Let go of what you thought motherhood would be like and be present to the unfolding of what actually 'is.' Be with it. Sit with it. Hold it, feel it, breathe it in. It's not here to hurt you. It's here to transform you.*"

—Brittany Chambers

I received a handmade Mother's Day card from Ryan this year. Why is that a big deal? Young children are encouraged, even required, in preschool and kindergarten to craft special mementos for their mothers in May. There is often a template to be followed, including a point-in-time handprint or photo surrounded by rhyming words to move Mom's emotions. But you see, Ryan is 21 years old. All on his own (or just maybe at the slight prompting of his sweet girlfriend), he used colored pencils, magic markers, and a glue stick to wish me a special day. The card came through the mail because he's not living at home this summer. He has an internship ahead of his senior year in college. He's preparing to leave my nest, and his ability to properly address an old-fashioned envelope is a further indication of his readiness. Where have 21 years gone?

It feels like a lifetime ago and only yesterday that Ryan joined me on this journey. I'm not the same person as I was then. His arrival shocked me, challenged me, and bettered me. I had 38 weeks of processing time, a healthy pregnancy, and a stocked nursery. As far as I could tell, I was blessed and set for success. You read my story, so you know there were some rough, scary, and dark days in my early motherhood. Writing that still feels like a risk. Am I unworthy of the privilege of motherhood? Who's going to report me to Child & Family Services? Will someone think I'm a bad mother because I'm honest about my struggles? It took me some time—and the support of other mothers—to grow into and embrace my new role in life. Once I did, I couldn't help going back for more.

I was pregnant with Michael by Ryan's first birthday, but then I slowed the pace a little, waiting four years before having Aedan. My boys are exactly what and whom I'm supposed to have. I recognize that I don't know what I'm missing, not having a daughter. Perhaps I'll have daughters-in-law one day. Regardless, my boys are my greatest achievements. Each was born to a different, constantly evolving mother and into a different family altogether. I grew an additional heart for each of them. I did things differently with each subsequent baby, according to what he needed, what I could give, and what I'd learned the last time around. By No.3, I was in a mindset more conducive to breastfeeding success, and I nursed Aedan for seven months. I'm grateful to have had that experience and I still have the occasional dream that I'm nursing a baby. It's a miraculous exchange that's hard to put words to. If we can indeed feed our babies and they are nourished, we have great fortune. I see beauty in choosing how we feed our babies based on our individual circumstances.

I formula-fed, I pumped, and I breastfed. Along the way, I wrote birth plans that both allowed and didn't allow epidurals. I worked full-time and had a nanny, I worked part-time and had the boys in daycare, and at a point, I didn't work for a paycheck at all. Now, I'm back to working full-time. Each boy turned out more than fine, despite my self-criticism and doubt. They're physically healthy, socially and emotionally sound, and most importantly, they're happy. We are entirely and deeply blessed, indeed. I've come to agree with Friedrich Nietzsche, the great philosopher, when he said, "You have your way. I have my way. As for the right way, the correct way, and the only way, it does not exist." I have great respect for how each of us does motherhood, whether we have a choice about it or not.

16 years after my last pregnancy, I still stop mid-stride to sneeze, oftentimes feeling a warm drop between my legs anyway. What a beautiful relic of my loves. I feel pangs of jealousy at the sight of a mother and her baby; I wish I could go back in time. And I'm still reading the books. I'm still searching for the right authority to guide me and tell me what to do according to the perfect parenting theory. Only recently did my research introduce me to the term "matrescence." Said simply, matrescence is anthropology's reference to the process of becoming a mother. It describes the all-encompassing physical, psychological, and emotional changes women go through on their journey to and through motherhood. Phew, the phenomenon has a name!

In our society, the celebration of new life is primarily centered around the baby's arrival. It's often glossed over that with the birth of a child, so too has a mother been born. Upon being born, she is charged with discovering who she is now and grappling with how that relates to who she once was and who she will eventually become. Matrescence has been largely unexplored in the medical community. More research is focused on the health and development of the baby than on the woman's identity transition. I've felt this on my own motherhood journey, and I bet you have, too.

 I survived. I more than survived, thanks to a postpartum support group. The honest sharing of experiences and non-judgmental idea exchange brought me out of the dark and into the light as a new mother. Ever since making that shift, I've contemplated how I might be a bright light for other women. How I might spread the messages I wish I'd been flooded with as a new mother. Now that my boys are older, I (finally) have the bandwidth to do so. I hope the stories within *Swaddled* have provided you solace, and I hope you'll read on to learn about additional opportunities for connection.

 I'll go out on a limb and say I believe I've been a good mother. Not a perfect mother, not even close. But a good one in the ways that count and in the sense that I've always been motivated by love. I hope my boys agree.

Closing

Your Story

"*In the wild, female elephants are known as fierce protectors. And when one of their sisters is suffering, they circle up around her. They close in tight, watch guard, and even kick dust around her to mask her vulnerable scent from predators. And yet, we are the same. This is who we are, and who we are meant to be for each other. Sometimes we're the ones in the middle. Sometimes we're the ones kicking up dust with fierce, fierce love. But the circle remains.*"

—The Festive Farm Company

I've heard variations on the juxtaposition of what new mothers were told they would need postpartum and what they actually needed. It goes something like this:

Expected needs: functional nursery, reliable stroller, newborn shoes, infant sleep schedule, diaper bag, six weeks' recovery, exercise program, birth control.

Actual needs: hot shower, non-judgmental advice, engaged partner, nutritious meals, guilt-free rest, diapers and more diapers of varied sizes, cleaning help, extra bed and crib sheets.

We have a gap! *Swaddled* is an attempt to close the gap

between expectations and reality—toward the goal of empowering women to be prepared and therefore, best positioned to enjoy the rapture of new motherhood while at the same time facing its challenges. I hope that in reading the stories of *Swaddled* you've received three clear messages: 1) You are not alone; 2) You are the perfect mother for your baby; and 3) Your life *will* come back to you.

Now that you've heard our stories, we want to hear yours!

Please, become part of the story and part of the movement. Together, we can normalize and celebrate: the joy, the struggle, the enormity, the confusion, and the sweet reward that is new motherhood. A sharing forum, a circle, saved me. Saved me from the depths of fear, loneliness, and comparison associated with new motherhood. My heart's dream is that this book and the *Swaddled* movement will do the same for you and countless other women. Let's lock arms and be fierce protectors of our sisters, as the elephants have demonstrated for us.

Let's bring our stories off the page, off the screen, and into life. *Swaddled* is a dynamic place where you yourself will be swaddled, and where you will have the opportunity to swaddle fellow mothers. While our stories are inevitably colored with different details, our core experience as mothers features many common threads. Let's weave those threads into a warm, cozy quilt to wrap each other in so much love. You'll find *Swaddled* at swaddledbysarah.com and via social media.

Lastly, as we deliver savory casseroles, fragrant flowers, and adorable accessories upon Baby's arrival, let's be sure to look the new mother in the eyes and ask how *she's* doing before we get understandably lost in oohing and aahing over Baby. Baby won't remember who held her, but Mama will always remember the care, compassion, and support she received.

Acknowledgments

"It's hard to wait for something you know might never happen; but it's even harder to give up when you know it's everything you want."

—Pranjal Sinha

The writing of Swaddled was influenced and supported by many. My authorship was seeded when my parents named me what they did (see dedication), and my deep desire to support new mothers sprouted upon finding my footing as Ryan's mother. Yet, defining that support took many years. Specifically, it took three goes at new motherhood studded with much experience, observation, and introspection sprinkled in along the way and in retrospect. My personal episodes of indescribable joy, deep valleys of doubt, and connection to other women brave enough to share the same came together and manifested as this book. The following individuals played key roles, and my gratitude is immeasurable.

Humbly and more briefly than you deserve, I thank you:

The ladies of this book for your courage and generosity in sharing your stories.

Dad for your voluminous and highly technical edits, but only upon my asking for them. You taught me more than I can quantify. Mom for your unwavering support and belief in me.

Ryan for making me a mother. Your gallantry stands out, and your resilience is remarkable. I have zero doubt that you will move mountains; you already have.

Michael for being my middle child who has never acted like a middle child. You entered the world efficiently and effectively, and you continue to live as such.

Aedan for being three of three. I didn't always know I needed you, but boy do I need you. You are a bright light in everything you do.

Monica for constantly monitoring this project and for willingly delving into every detail like it was your own to wrangle.

Lisa for being my friend and sister since 1992. Enough said.

Aimee for always cheering for me and encouraging me no matter what. You see what's in the stars.

Crissy for hanging with me since way before we were thinking about *this* kind of stuff. May we continue to make family memories.

Brie for meeting me where I was that day at "Transitions to Motherhood." It's impossible to reflect on my early months as a mother without thinking of the understanding and acceptance you offered me.

Sheryl for being the best writing buddy turned dear friend a girl could hope for. We've covered it all on our calls and in our texts, from accountability and time management to preservation of sanity and support of our dependents.

Karolina for being my first life coach and for helping me see the necessity of writing this book as part of my purpose here. Your work is invaluable to so many.

Sara for living and breathing your knowing that stories change lives. Your guidance and the support of Thought Leader Academy were my framework in completing this project.

Mary for your loving and patient editing brilliance. You've ridden this wave with me through multiple variations of this book and never (audibly) laughed at me.

Susie for bringing this book into the world! I will forever be grateful for the chance to work with you, the book doula. Your wisdom, professionalism, and pure effectiveness are precious and rare.

Claudine for bringing my vision to reality by way of your unique talent and dedication. Your artistry transformed my thoughts and words into a visual hug for our readership.

Last but not least, Doug for being the other half of our children's DNA and for being a dedicated and loving husband and father. We move quickly and have been incredibly blessed in what has come our way.

Playlist

Swaddled
"Never Gonna Let You Down," Colbie Caillat

Epigraph
"Next Thing You Know," Jordan Davis

Preface
"Nobody Told Me," John Lennon

1. **My Story**
"This Is Me," Keala Settle

2. **Danielle**
"The Fighter," Keith Urban

3. **Monica**
"Higher Love," Steve Winwood

4. **Aimee**
"These Are Days," 10,000 Maniacs

5. **Sara**
"Ain't No Mountain High Enough," Marvin Gaye and Tammi Terrell

6. **Sheryl**
"Hallelujah," Jeff Buckley

7. **Brie**
   "Love Don't," Nathaniel Rateliff

8. **Meredith**
   "I Hope You Dance," LeeAnn Womack

9. **Nicole**
   "Calling All Angels," Train

10. **Cora**
    "Shot at the Night," The Killers

11. **Amanda**
    "Be Here Now," Ray LaMontagne

12. **Ashlee**
    "Mother and Child Reunion," Paul Simon

Epilogue
"Bright Side of the Road," Van Morrison

Closing
"You Raise Me Up," Josh Groban

Acknowledgments
"Hall of Fame," The Script

Apple Music

Spotify

About the Author

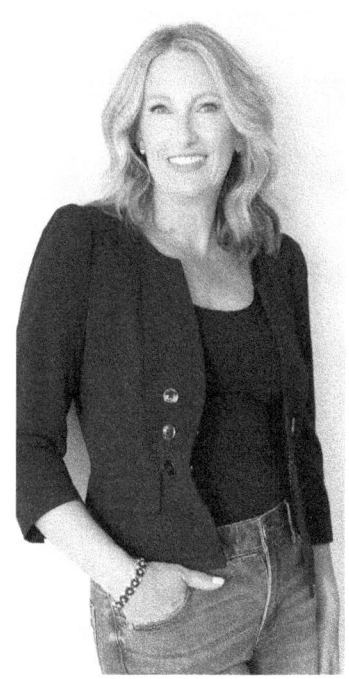

Elizabeth Sarah Cassidy is passionate about supporting new mothers as they enter one of the most remarkable passages of their lifetime. For as statistically common an experience as motherhood is, Sarah finds that truthful conversation about its nuances remains muted. She encourages transparent looks at the transition to honor the rainbow of experiences amongst women. Sarah lives outside of Chicago with her husband, two four-leggeds, and whichever of her three young men happen to be home.

swaddledbysarah.com

www.ingramcontent.com/pod-product-compliance
Lightning Source LLC
Chambersburg PA
CBHW020538030426
42337CB00013B/891